T0049340

Praise for *Yoga Wise*

"This book is a privilege to read, to contemplate, and to own. It delivers on the promise that all authors should fulfill for their readers: it educates, inspires, and informs. Chanson's work broadens the reader's mindset and reaches into the heart, facilitating change. The effect on the individual is personal growth. The impact on society is hope." **—Julie Ryan McGue, author of the award-winning memoir *Twice a Daughter: A Search for Identity, Family, and Belonging***

"Seasoned with personal experience, directed practices, and ancient teachings, this is a book of transformation in daily doses that is begging to be read, reflected on, and taken to heart. The end of 365 days will find the reader with a heart more open, a will more disciplined, and surprised by the potency of small consistent effort." **—Deborah Adele, author of *The Yamas & Niyamas: Exploring Yoga's Ethical Practice***

YOGA
· W · I · S · E ·

About the Author

Molly Chanson, MA, (Milwaukee, WI) has been practicing yoga for more than thirty years and completed her teacher training at the renowned Kripalu Center for Yoga and Health in Massachusetts. Molly is an educator, writer, and entrepreneur who taught writing and international English courses at Columbia College in Chicago for fourteen years. Molly is the founder of The Practice, a yearlong yoga course online that teaches the physical and ethical practices of yoga as a path to transformation. Molly's first book, *Fallen Star: A Return to Self through the Eight Limbs of Yoga* (April 2022), is a memoir through sobriety and divorce and how the tenets of yoga can be utilized to overcome any adversity.

MOLLY CHANSON, MA

YOGA
WISE

365 Days of
Yoga-Inspired Teachings to
Transform Your Life

Llewellyn Publications | Woodbury, MN

FIRST EDITION
First Printing, 2023

Book design by Christine Ha
Cover design by Cassie Willett

Llewellyn Publications is a registered trademark of Llewellyn Worldwide Ltd.

Library of Congress Cataloging-in-Publication Data (Pending)
Names: Chanson, Molly, author.
Title: Yoga wise : 365 days of yoga-inspired teachings to transform your
   life / Molly Chanson.
Description: First edition. | Woodbury, MN : Llewellyn Worldwide, ltd,
   2023. | Includes bibliographical references. | Summary: "Explore
   meditation and yoga poses designed to help you align with your truth,
   find your purpose, and walk through the fire until you transform,
   gaining a new sense of Self"— Provided by publisher.
Identifiers: LCCN 2022058749 (print) | LCCN 2022058750 (ebook) | ISBN
   9780738773827 | ISBN 9780738773889 (ebook)
Subjects: LCSH: Yoga. | Meditation. | Self-actualization (Psychology)
Classification: LCC B132.Y6 C553 2023 (print) | LCC B132.Y6 (ebook) | DDC
   181/.45—dc23/eng/20230211
LC record available at https://lccn.loc.gov/2022058749
LC ebook record available at https://lccn.loc.gov/2022058750

Llewellyn Worldwide Ltd. does not participate in, endorse, or have any authority or responsibility concerning private business transactions between our authors and the public.

All mail addressed to the author is forwarded but the publisher cannot, unless specifically instructed by the author, give out an address or phone number.

Any internet references contained in this work are current at publication time, but the publisher cannot guarantee that a specific location will continue to be maintained. Please refer to the publisher's website for links to authors' websites and other sources.

Llewellyn Publications
A Division of Llewellyn Worldwide Ltd.
2143 Wooddale Drive
Woodbury, MN 55125-2989
www.llewellyn.com

Printed in the United States of America

Other Books by Molly Chanson

Fallen Star:
A Return to Self through the Eight Limbs of Yoga
(Shanti Arts, 2022)

For my sister, Anne,
the wisest, bravest, truest person I know.

Contents

Disclaimer

The information provided in this book is for educational and informational purposes only and to be used as a self-guided self-help tool for your own personal use and discernment. The author is not a medical or mental health professional and is not able to diagnose or treat any disease or mental/emotional issue. The information provided in this book regarding body, weight, addictions, health, spirituality, or relationships is not meant to be absolute, nor a substitute for medical or mental health advice provided by a professional. This book offers suggestions to support you on your own transformative journey; however, individual results cannot be predicted or guaranteed. While there is scientific research to support yoga's effects on the mind and body, every individual has their own experience and is expected to practice self-care and personal responsibility when beginning their own yoga practice. Information throughout this book is based on the author's personal experience as well as the experience of other authors and yoga instructors who have educated and inspired the author along her journey. The author shares her true experience and knowledge on the subject of yoga as a resource only, and it is to be applied to your current circumstance as you see fit.

Introduction

I got sober and divorced in the same year. It was a complete undoing of life as I knew it, and I was forced to surrender to an unknown path ahead. It was daunting, but I felt a bit of relief from the self-imposed abuse that had taken place over my lifetime. My go-to behaviors of perfectionism, bulimia, and numbing, rather than feeling, eventually caught up with me. Yet I sensed hope. I sensed support from the Universe that I was on the right path. I glimpsed freedom from the cage and possibility for my future.

On the outside, my life looked pretty good—the house, husband, two kids, career. Inside, I was on fire. My soul knew something was not right. In yoga, the *subtle body* is the part of us that knows. It is our wise inner teacher, our gut, and our intuition. We can have a beautiful exterior. We can piece together the perfect life and yet feel unfulfilled. We are taught that if we gather the right people and things to surround us, we will be happy. Yoga teaches us that true happiness and fulfillment comes from within, and they are achieved by a "right" way of daily practice. *Right* doesn't mean "perfect." It means we show up as we are. We show up humble, curious, and compassionate. We show up brave and ready.

When my life collapsed, my yoga mat became my sacred space for healing and self-care. No matter how much my insides were in turmoil over my marriage, my addiction, or my lost sense of Self,

I showed up to my daily practice. Sometimes, the postures were horrible, and sometimes, they flowed. Sometimes, my body let go, and I experienced a reprieve from the chaos at home. Other times, my mind chattered and berated about how I had screwed everything up so badly. The funny thing is, I didn't even know why or how I chose yoga. I have done yoga since I was fifteen and, from the beginning, have always been pulled toward the poses and the lessons I received. Yoga is not exercise, nor is it therapy. Yoga is not complete stillness, and yet it's not constant doing. All I know is during a time when my mind was lost, my body dying, and my soul on fire, I chose yoga. I chose the comfort of my mat and sought answers from my own body.

I learned that yoga is much more than asana, the physical practice. While I believe our body is a starting point and the gateway to all healing, yoga is also beliefs, sacred rituals, breath, focus, commitment, self-study, and self-love. Yoga holds the wisdom and the practices to get through life's challenges and to discover who you are in the process. Happiness and fulfillment are attained when we live the life we were meant to live. Not for anyone else—not for our parents or society—but for ourselves.

Whatever conflict you are faced with today, whatever healing needs to take place, I urge you to take the time to turn inward. Rather than seek answers outside yourself, in another person, job, location, or possession, begin with your own heart. Yoga tends to the physical body as well as the soul, and before we can know what we want, we have to know who we are. Maybe you expected your life to turn out differently. Maybe you are in the middle of a difficult experience you never thought you'd be facing. Maybe your past is revealing itself. Whether you already have a consistent yoga practice or have never done yoga, this book takes you through a transformational process with yoga philosophy as the foundation and the practice for life. This book is for everybody, regardless of yoga experience, and gives you lessons that you can apply to your own being and circumstance. These practices support your inward journey in order to be free from stories and experiences of the past, to access unconditional love for yourself and others, to redefine your roles and expectations, and to live purposefully and fulfilled as your authentic Self.

The practice starts with one day, one quiet morning, and one quick read to ponder. *Simple, right?* Then you complete the same ritual the next day and the next. The ritual starts off clunky but soon becomes sacred and builds. Then one day you realize—something is different … *I'm different.*

You commit to your practice, which isn't perfect, but it's something you come back to. It's something in your chaos that keeps you tethered, not to the past but to your present—to the right now.

As you show up for yourself, you become aware of how you feel and what comes up. There is a deep and profound inner teacher we often dismiss in our busy day-to-day. It's like we are treading water to the point of exhaustion, and when we finally let go, stop all the paddling, gasping, and effort and simply observe our circumstance, we realize that we float a little easier.

The events that break us open are the same events that bring us to healing—and not just healing from those events but maybe a healing that is long overdue. It is a healing of our soul and a redirecting of our energy, a transformation into who we were always meant to be. This transformation happens when we are brave enough to remain present. It happens when we are so desperate and so out of solutions that all we can do is surrender to the present and observe our inner sensations—maybe for the first time.

We stop resisting and railing against the moment. We stop asking ourselves: *Why now? Why this? Why me?* We stop trying to figure everything out.

When all the reasons, excuses, and blame have been exhausted, we are finally convinced we must take care of ourselves. We get up early to meditate like we have promised we would do so many times before. We make time like we should have all along. We buy the yoga mat we've had in our virtual shopping cart, and we make space. Finally, it is time.

If I had not been through very difficult times, I would not have the faith, gratitude, or presence I have today. I would not believe in myself. I would not know my strength or my resilience. I would not know the freedom of listening to my own heart.

Here is the big secret: When we go through difficult times, we are forced to operate on an amount of surrender we never knew we were capable of. We are forced to let go absolutely, which feels foreign and unnatural. But once we get the hang of it, we wonder why we ever struggled so much in the first place. Why are we grasping? Why are we making things hard? If your world is a mess, or if you feel like everything is upside down, pay attention. There is a nugget of wisdom about who you are and how you operate in every single aspect of your life. And once you start the practice of coming back to yourself, instead of seeking answers outside, I believe that not only is there nothing you cannot overcome, but there is nothing you desire that you will not accomplish.

I invite you to read a page of this book every day as part of a daily practice. It does not matter what date in the year you begin this book; start at the beginning, with day 1. In the case of a leap year, there is a 366th day, which can be read at the end to account for the extra day. The chapters cover twelve practices, which I have based on yoga philosophy, psychology, twelve-step recovery, and my own experience. Some days invite you to journal, meditate, or do a yoga pose. The yoga and meditation instructions are in italicized text to indicate this is an invitation to practice. While I offer accessible cues for each posture, it may help to look up the poses online to get an idea of where you are going if you are new to yoga. For the guided meditations, it will help to read through them first before closing your eyes or to record them so you can listen. You are welcome to have a special journal dedicated to your practice and to use it to write from the prompts or to reflect on the readings.

The chapters are meant to be digested in order and to build on one another. It will not take the entire book to experience shifts and changes in your body, mind, and heart. Each day, your practice will grow with you and you with it. At the end of the book, you will arrive transformed with a new sense of Self and a deep appreciation for who you are and where you've been. The answers you seek are within you. Let's access them—one day at a time.

PRACTICE 1
Cleansing (Saucha)

Our first practice is *saucha*. *Saucha* is Sanskrit for "cleansing" and "purity," and it is one of the five niyamas (the five sacred observances) on the Eight-Limbed Path of Yoga. We cleanse the body with hygiene, water, and healthy foods. We cleanse the mind from false beliefs and old stories. We cleanse our physical spaces, our habits, and our relationships. We observe the practice of saucha as a way to open space and to align with our true Self—our best Self. To practice saucha, we will focus on getting lighter physically and mentally. We will create space for our senses in order to release stuck energy, acknowledge old wounds, and begin new habits instead of repeating the less healthy behaviors that weigh us down.

DAY 1

What does it mean to harmonize with your true Self? What does it mean to harmonize with life and the Universe?

In art, when a color aligns with another, it is called toning. The colors balance each other out and harmonize. They work together. They make one another more beautiful than if they stayed alone. Likewise, our body tones and aligns when we take care of it, when we strengthen certain muscles and pay attention to the food we eat.

Cleansing can look like eliminating food and drink that is bad for our bodies, drinking more water, using a neti pot, rinsing our face before bed, brushing our teeth, yoga, stillness, and breath.

Like our physical body, our soul tones and aligns when we rid the emotional Self of unnecessary heaviness such as worry, anxiety, resentment, or fear. Carrying the heaviness of the past or junk in the present leaves no room to breathe or see clearly.

Ask yourself, what needs cleansing in or around you at this moment? Is there physical clutter dragging you down or emotional weight you no longer need to carry? Are there habits you would like to let go? We will dive deeper into these questions as we observe and practice the ancient ritual of saucha.

DAY 2

The practice of cleansing starts in the body. If you've ever eaten too much rich or unhealthy food, you know the sensation of wanting to cleanse. You might call this "dieting," but the practice of saucha means so much more than trying to lose weight. Saucha includes eliminating food and drink that is bad for our bodies; eating cleansing foods, such as greens and vegetables; drinking more water; brushing our teeth; and other parts of a hygiene routine. It's likely you already practice saucha without realizing it. In yoga, the purpose of a healthy, cleansed body is not about appearance. The purpose of cleansing is to rid ourselves of the physical and emotional heaviness that prevents us from seeing ourselves clearly. When we lift the weight, we open space to listen.

Ayurveda is considered a sister practice to yoga, and it is a way of healing the entire body, including how we eat, sleep, exercise, and rest. Related to saucha, ayurveda teaches that the body needs to be cleansed after every sleep. Physical gunk collected while we rested should be removed and cleared out before we begin our new day. Consider your normal waking routine, such as brushing your teeth, rinsing your face, or drinking a glass of water. Begin to see this time as sacred. Acknowledge that you are participating in the practice of saucha, the ancient yogic principle of cleansing, and this daily practice will seep into all other areas of your life.

DAY 3

How we treat our body provides much insight into how we treat our Self. Being "clean" from a physical standpoint is the first step to purifying deeper, less obvious messes. By practicing a waking ritual of saucha, we acknowledge our body as sacred and set the tone for our day. In addition to cleaning the body, we are also signaling to the emotional Self that yesterday has ended, and today is a new day. We remove the gunk from the past and begin again.

Beyond what you already do, here are some cleansing tips upon waking:

+ First thing, drink a glass of warm water
+ Brush your teeth and scrape your tongue
+ Rinse your eyes, nose, and mouth
+ Use a neti pot
+ Practice some breath or gentle yoga
+ Practice silence—try not speaking, turning on the TV, or looking at your phone first thing in the morning
+ Set aside time to be still, meditate, or journal

Like all new beginnings, ease gently in. Create space before charging ahead with work and the to-do list. Adding these new cleansing rituals to the start of your day should help lighten feelings of being overwhelmed, busyness, and even fear about what the day will bring.

DAY 4
Tadasana (Mountain Pose)

Stand with your feet hip-distance apart or even a little wider. Be comfortable with effort in the legs but with soft knees. Ground yourself through the feet and breathe. Tadasana is a standing posture that allows us to tune in while feeling strong and supported. Position your pelvis in a spot that feels neutral, without your low back swaying in or out. Stand with a straight spine and lengthen through the crown of your head. Release your shoulders back and down and open your arms to the sides.

Close your eyes and breathe. Notice the breath as if you are noticing it for the first time. Maybe you haven't paid attention to how the breath moves and feels. This is a practice in observing; there is no technique and nothing to control or do. Examine the breath exactly as it is on this day. Observe the inhale through your nose and then the exhale that arrives after. Notice where the breath travels after it enters the nose—belly, ribs, and upper chest. Notice the rising and falling of your heart space. After some breaths, bring your attention to your feet. Notice the soles of your feet on the earth. Feel the surface beneath them. Observe if you are rocking slightly, shifting weight from one area of the feet to another.

Mountain pose cultivates the inner witness; we observe our body exactly as it is in this posture. Possibly, we can then practice being this nonjudgmental witness in other areas of our life. By giving the body stillness and our acknowledgment, we offer ourselves space before running into the day.

DAY 5

When we cleanse our body through breath and movement and cleanse the mind through inquiry and meditation, we open space for truth to enter. Imagine you have a closet jammed full of clothes, shoes, and other stuff. It would be hard to find anything inside the mess. Practicing saucha is a great way to prepare our body and mind to receive the awakening consciousness within us. Creating space is powerful. If we are full of "stuff," we can't hear or experience the truth of our being.

When I am weighed down emotionally, my body responds with impatience, fatigue, or even illness. My brain feels foggy and confused. I can't decide whether to go to the store, do laundry, or sit down and write. I feel pulled in many directions and am unable to focus. Confusion and a sense of being overwhelmed is my body alerting me that I have become cluttered. There's no room to breathe, let alone act in accordance with my true Self. There is only enough left in me to react, and reacting may get a person by for a bit, but it's no way to thrive. Focusing on saucha and some cleansing rituals, such deep breaths, simple postures, and good nutrition, helps us get rid of confusion and the sensation of being overwhelmed and creates space for our most productive Self. When your mind and your day seem jammed with stuff and busyness, eliminate the outside distractions, even for a few minutes, and make space for yourself.

DAY 6

Cultivating the witness is a foundational practice to all of yoga. Rather than behave from a place of forcing or pushing, we observe our body and our actions with compassion and nonjudgment. At the heart of yoga, we are kind to ourselves; we witness rather than critique. As we embark on the practice of saucha, keep in mind that cleansing is a sacred ritual. From washing your face in the morning to twisting the body in a pose to clearing out space for your practice, yoga brings us to a place of inquiry where we ask questions rather than demand clear answers.

On day 4, we practiced observing the breath while standing in tadasana. Just like we can notice the body as a witness, we can also observe thoughts and emotions. Saucha refers to purifying the physical body as well as our emotional self. While cleansing the body may be familiar, it gets slightly more complex when we dive into our mind. You can start to examine your emotional purity by asking yourself some questions. I invite you to journal around these questions as a nonjudgmental witness and see what comes up:

+ What load am I carrying that I want to lighten?
+ What thoughts feel *heavy*?
+ Is there something or someone I am holding on to from the past?
+ Am I letting past regret or future worry get in the way of the present moment?
+ What do I fear? What makes me not want to get out of bed in the morning?

DAY 7

After a few days with a mindful waking routine and some brief moments asking yourself what it is you are carrying, some interesting insights might be arriving for you. Trust it all—trust yourself. To engage in the practice of yoga, which includes self-awareness, you must accept what comes up in order to learn. If you have something nagging at you to be addressed, trust that. If the idea of cleansing out old junk scares you, whether it be a drawer in your kitchen or an emotion in your soul, trust that. It means this process is revealing truth to you.

Start small and continue to observe. Get to the junk drawer; open the hall closet; clear a corner for your mat. Notice how cleaning out spaces in your home also opens space in your being. Notice that you feel lighter, more intentional, and more present.

Now, ask yourself: *"If this physical stuff is making me feel heavy, what emotional junk am I not cleaning out? How would I feel if I did?"*

Return to the question from day 6: *What thoughts feel heavy?*

Human beings are excellent at distraction. We distract ourselves from feeling pain or discomfort, and after years of doing so, the emotions build up. We stay busy out of responsibility and obligation but also out of not wanting to feel. We turn on the TV, eat or drink, or focus our attention elsewhere. To practice saucha is to begin to let yourself feel. Don't be surprised if uncomfortable sensations arise.

DAY 8

We get so comfortable carrying things from our past, we might not even realize they have become cumbersome and detrimental. Just like extra weight on the body, the heaviness does not happen overnight. The process is gradual, pound by pound, and our body adapts slowly over time. It can be difficult to get rid of a cherished possession in order to make space, and we cling to old experiences in the body the same way. We cling to them because they are familiar. We hold on because the fear of losing something is greater than whether or not we want it anymore.

Familiar possessions and familiar behaviors keep us hostage and therefore deserve assessment. It's worth it to look at our outer surroundings as well as our inner landscape in order to determine what needs clearing. Relationships are another area where the familiar can override what is healthy or beneficial to our current well-being and circumstance. We put up with someone's unhealthy behaviors—or even abuse—and the added stress is insidious. We have let something happen over time, and now, we wonder why we feel so heavy and stuck.

Just as the heaviness arrived, little by little, we can chip away at it. We can clean out the messy drawer and then tackle the entire basement. If we have spent too long refusing our own needs, we can slowly start to take care of ourselves again by introducing cleansing rituals that are good for our body and our heart. Slowly, we will become stronger until the weight doesn't feel so impossible to remove.

DAY 9

When I got divorced, I moved twice in the same year. While moving, I couldn't believe the stuff I was holding on to from my marriage, which was probably preventing me from moving on in a new life and a new relationship.

I had all of our wedding china. Despite having no need for the wedding gift, I felt obligated to keep it. I lugged the dishes, saucers, teacups, and serving ware with me. Every dish and cup was kept in white protective containers. And that's where they stayed. I never used the dishes or even displayed them.

With each move, I watched myself carry the china gently into the car and then unload it, box by box. On the last move, I found a high cabinet above the refrigerator, grabbed the step stool, and started climbing up. I strained to lift the first heavy box above my head, thinking this would be the last time I'd have to deal with these useless dishes. All of a sudden, my mind screamed, *This is crazy!* The drop-off at the donation center was one of the most freeing moments since my divorce.

What are you dragging around that you no longer want? What are you holding on to out of guilt, obligation, or just because it's the way things have always been? Today, what can you do to let it go and be free?

DAY 10

Sanskrit words have many definitions, and another meaning of *saucha* is "purity." *Purity* doesn't mean "perfection," as we might think. Purity actually refers to presence and truth. Can you accept what *is* right now?

As the witness, can you observe your uncomfortable emotions with nonjudgment? Can you accept difficult sensations, such as anxiety, sadness, resentment, anger, or fear? Your feelings are valid, and expecting them to disappear is the opposite of practicing saucha.

What saucha asks us to practice is accepting these emotions as they are in the moment. Saucha also asks us to accept people, places, and things as they are in the moment instead of wishing they were different. We cannot manufacture a pure situation or relationship. We make a situation pure through our acceptance of it.

One of the most challenging practices for me has been to accept my whole Self as I am right now—not who I want to be in the future but *right now*. Accepting ourselves as we are does not mean we don't want to change and grow. It means we are not critical or guilt ridden for where we are today.

If we think of saucha this way—purity in what already *is*—we release the heaviness of wishing something were different. Saucha is as much about the present moment and acceptance of what is true right now as it is about cleansing, decluttering, and lightening. Loading ourselves up with guilt, shame, regret, and expectation is heavy on our souls and makes any progress difficult.

DAY 11

The idea of cleansing has been churning in your mind for several days now. It's time to set an intention about what you would like to welcome in. Having pondered some of the previous questions this week, where is your body leading you? When we trust our intuition, rather than an outsider's advice, we find that we already know what we need. We know our deepest longings and desires, but we are distracted by society's image or a friend's well-meaning words.

Accept that you already know what you desire, and take a few minutes to get still, either in meditation or with a journal. If nothing comes, ask yourself, "*What do I crave? What in my life is heavy?*" Consider your intention to be something you want to welcome in, such as love, strength, community, healing. Your intention might look like this: *I welcome in* _____.

When the answer arrives, trust it. Write it down or secure the intention in your mind. Try not to force a solution or any action at all. Simply acknowledge and accept. Even if the words or names don't make sense, let your body feel and experience their essence—their subtle meaning on your heart.

Feel free to write your intention on a sticky note and place it somewhere you will read it every day. This will secure your intention and remind you of your desire.

DAY 12

When you become aware of your intention, check in with your body for any next steps. You might instinctively redecorate a room in your home or call a friend and speak some much-needed words. You might dedicate an hour in your day to yoga or to preparing a healthy meal.

Once your intention is set, you may feel pulled to take action somewhere in your routine, your home, or another part of your life. With every small action forward, guided by your desire, you will begin to feel lighter, more open, and less afraid. You will begin the journey of stepping into yourself and your truth by taking small steps toward a larger purpose.

The practice is a process. Cleansing is a process. Grant yourself grace and compassion as you explore your own relationship to cleansing and purity. As you clean out and declutter, know you are moving forward, but do not be discouraged when you slip back. Ride the waves, and return to your intention. Rather than view your intention as a goal or a must-do list, something to be checked off and never thought of again, observe the root. Try not to tackle the intention from the branches by assuming you know the steps needed to achieve an end result. Instead, bear witness to your deepest desire—the way you want to feel (or not feel) once the intention comes to light.

Clearing space—inside and around you—takes an amount of trust and invites in many possibilities. Stay open because possibilities are infinite, and something you never dreamed of might present itself.

DAY 13

To begin a practice of anything, we start slow and awkward. We accept that we don't know yet what the practice will bring. All we know is that by engaging in the practice, more will be revealed. The practice takes commitment, consistency, and courage. We try and we fall short. We let go and we take it back. We become aware of something we want to be rid of, but we understand that nothing can be done in an instant. Donating my wedding china offered me a glimpse of letting go and was a step forward, but the progress didn't mean my marriage and my divorce did not still affect me. I backtrack all the time into old thinking and patterns, and I need to return to my practice, again and again, in order to actually be free.

To practice saucha is to explore our body and our emotions. We make space in order to listen. By asking questions, we open ourselves up to receive insight without the violent force of manipulation or the disappointing fallout of expectation. Saucha expands our willingness as well as our trust. We continue the practice even if we don't notice immediate results. We continue because we know that undoing weeks, months, or years of any learned behavior takes gentleness and self-compassion. If, at any point, you start to feel discouraged, come back to your intention. Remember the heart of your reason, and know you are making progress. If, at any point, your intention shifts or changes, write that in your journal as well. None of this needs to be a straight line, and anything arriving right now is meant for you.

DAY 14

When we discuss saucha and the idea of purity, remember that being pure does not mean being perfect. A big part of saucha is clearing out what happened yesterday in order to be present with what is today. This refers to our efforts from years ago as well as efforts from the day before. Notice your expectations. Maybe you started reading this book and put a lot of pressure on yourself to have a perfect waking routine.

If our effort wasn't perfect yesterday or last week, we don't need to let it paralyze us to the point of giving up or being overly critical. Like waking and cleansing the body of junk acquired while we slept, we can also rinse away our efforts of yesterday and begin again. Saucha, and all of yoga, is a constant practice and a constant return. To practice purity does not mean we *only* eat healthy food, or we *always* say the right thing, or we *always* get to our yoga mat. By accepting ourselves where we are, that we are not perfect, we cleanse away emotions, such as guilt, sadness, regret, and self-loathing, that serve no purpose for today's efforts.

As you continue to lighten your body and mind, as you continue to tone through yoga and movement, as you continue to clear out physical space in your home, be mindful of the space you are creating to experience the presence, newness, and possibility of today.

DAY 15

In addition to our home, body, and mind, we can also practice saucha in our relationships. In the same way we practice accepting our emotions, saucha asks us to accept people, places, and things as they are in the moment instead of wishing they were different.

It's very common to think if a person or circumstance in your life were different, you would feel better—happier, more fulfilled, at peace. But yoga teaches us that we cannot achieve our inner longings, our deepest desires, from the outside-in. Changing a person or relationship will not automatically bring us what we want unless we also do the work of changing from our inside-out. When we accept a person or situation as is, we are able to make the healthiest decisions for ourselves.

Acceptance does not mean we don't have choices. We can stay or leave a relationship, and we can set boundaries and decide whom to let into our lives. Acceptance doesn't mean we allow abuse or unhealthy situations, but rather than try and change the other person, we recognize where we have control and where we don't. Often, we believe if someone else would change, then we would change. It is the opposite. Change yourself, your behaviors, and your reactions, and those around you will either fall away or shift to meet you.

DAY 16

Practicing silence is a great way to explore our inner Self. In terms of saucha, silence grants the opportunity to be present with what is while free from day-to-day distraction. You can practice silence over several days, but if this is not convenient, being silent in the morning, while eating, or even while holding space with others can offer much insight through normal activities and interactions.

During my yoga teacher training, we entered silence for three days as an inquiry practice. We were encouraged to not speak, use our phones, or go on the internet. The practice was awkward at first, but after a few hours, my body settled in. I learned the intimacy of a friendly smile rather than a conversation. I noticed the taste and texture of food as it entered my mouth and began digesting. I quickly learned how much outside noise acted as a barrier to my inner world. I realized parts of myself that had been nagging for my attention, but I couldn't hear the whispers amid the hum of daily life.

Consider where you can welcome silence into your life. Observe your reaction when you can't talk back, or when you want to scroll through your phone, but it is not an option. Observe how much these seemingly normal activities block access to your gut and your intuition. Internal chatter gets much louder when we are silent. You might notice harsh thoughts or critical ways you speak to yourself. The practice of silence is not to judge how we are, but it can lend much insight into the noisy mind, and you might start to appreciate, even crave, periods of thoughtful reflection.

DAY 17

Whether you realize it or not, your practice so far is very brave. Digging into yourself and asking what needs to be cleared out is courageous work. Most people won't even go there. Most people are very comfortable with a lifetime of buildup and clutter. It gets to the point that they are so overwhelmed by their possessions, they have no room or time to look at themselves, which is fine because looking at oneself is hard! Unlike physical objects, which can be tossed out or dropped off, never to be seen again, emotional clutter usually needs more attention. Sometimes, we clean out a pattern, belief, or behavior only to watch it resurface. In fact, you may find the same relationship or behavior pattern showing up a lot once you become aware of it. The good news about a pattern resurfacing is that it means you are that much closer to releasing it. When something shows up, it is because our awareness and, therefore, our willingness has grown. The pattern has become uncomfortable to the point that we no longer accept it as normal. Once we start to believe that we no longer need to tolerate the pattern, we open up to new ideas and possibilities—new ways of being—and this willingness gives us the courage to keep going.

Many times during a yoga practice, uncomfortable sensations arrive to meet us. Resist the urge to push these emotions away. As you allow yourself to feel, awareness grows. As awareness grows, willingness becomes more accessible. One day, that pesky pattern won't pull at you so tightly, and you'll realize creating space to look at yourself was indeed brave.

DAY 18

Imagine cleaning out an old basement, one that has been the dumping spot for everything you don't want to organize or deal with. Over the years, the space has become darker, smaller, and more suffocating. No one even wants to go down there; it's too painful. You don't know why, but your heart speeds up at the top of the stairs. Scared, you close the door on the basement and vow to touch it all on another day—when you have more time and a better game plan.

Having scheduled off a chunk of a day and feeling hopeful and motivated, you decide to make a start. You open the door, tread down the stairs, and start shuffling items and organizing contents. But quickly, you see you are creating more mess, more chaos, rather than less. Opening tucked-away boxes reveals more stuff than you had remembered. More dirt gets churned up that was otherwise hidden quietly in the corners. Partway through you wonder, *"Am I in too deep? This looks worse than when I started. Maybe I should have left it all alone?"*

Cleaning is a messy job, and things might look worse before they look better.

Emotional cleaning is no different. We don't see the benefit until near the end of the process. As you pick up and dust off your emotional Self, know that discomfort as a result of churning is normal. Be kind to yourself along the way. It's okay to take breaks. It's okay to back off. It's okay to shut the basement door and pick up where you left off next weekend.

DAY 19

While cleansing, try not to berate yourself when something ugly or dark arrives. This means you're uncovering something meaningful, and you have the choice to keep it, donate it, repurpose it, or throw it away.

The practice of saucha does not require a complete undoing all at once. Saucha is a life practice so that any buildup is not too daunting. As we clear out bad habits, false beliefs, and thoughts that no longer serve us, we are able to keep a clean house. We don't have overwhelming emotional projects because we've been mindfully clearing space along the way. We get used to feeling clear and unconfused. When something does block our energy, we notice, and we take care of it promptly. With daily practice, we get used to the sensation of a pure mind and heart, and it's noticeable when something nags at us.

There may be lots of clutter at the beginning of cleansing, but over time, once the larger issues have been addressed and excavated, saucha becomes a daily habit. Purity becomes our character rather than such a deliberate discipline.

At the end, we are happy with the clean basement or difficult project. We admire the organized shelves and the fact that we know where everything is. We can see the floor. We can see our stuff. We can see the transformation. We promise not to neglect the basement again so we don't have such a time-consuming and painful task. And what about when the basement does inevitably get cluttered and overlooked? Yoga teaches that we compassionately—and without judgment—bring ourselves back and begin again.

DAY 20

Human beings are born to create. Creativity exists inside each of our souls and is not limited to "the arts" such as painting, drawing, or music. Creation is our soul's expression of the moment, and therefore our anchor to the present. During our creative process, we access and acknowledge parts of ourselves from deep within. We honor our truth, and we are able to be present rather than inside a story in our mind. As a result of our focus, the mind is being cleansed and purified. Unnecessary distractions slip away, and we are brought to absolute attention.

Take a minute to think about the creative expressions that bring you joy: cooking, gardening, painting, photography, writing, dancing, crafting, sewing…

I have a feeling you create every day, even if you don't consider yourself an artist. You decorate a home, you grow a garden, you write a poem. Do not underestimate the process of creation in order to bring you to presence. When I write, I go to another place, unable to worry or be attached to my problems. I know cooks who get blissfully lost in the stirring of risotto. I know potters who find pure contentment as they touch and mold the soft clay.

To access our creativity is to access our soul. When we bring forth something from our heart's desire, we acknowledge the part of ourselves that needs no effort or explanation. We don't need someone's permission or approval. We don't create for fame or fortune. We create because it is part of who we are. And when we behave within our truth, we cultivate a present mind and a pure heart.

DAY 21

Do you feel a little lighter? Maybe a little freer? Has cleansing become part of your ritual and your intention? It takes twenty-one days to create a new habit—one that will "stick" and become less like a chore. At this stage, reflect on what it has been like to bring your awareness to the practice of truth, acceptance, and cleansing.

At the beginning of this practice, we asked a few questions:

- What load am I carrying that I want to lighten?
- What thoughts feel *heavy*?
- Is there something or someone I am holding on to from the past?
- Am I letting past regret or future worry get in the way of the present moment?
- What do I fear? What makes me not want to get out of bed in the morning?

The practice of yoga and meditation is a great way to clear distracting energy and open your body and your spirit to receive intuitive wisdom. If emotions have been coming up, that's because you are making space for them to arrive. You are becoming aware of your true Self, the part of you that has longed to be acknowledged.

We spend a lot of time staying busy and distracted in our day-to-day, so if you find you are noticing more about your body and emotions, that is good! Be proud of all you have done in a very short time.

DAY 22

There may be lots of activity happening as you practice saucha. New morning routines and new yoga schedules. You may feel busy with tasks in the home, such as cleaning out space and reorganizing rooms, but cleansing is also about stillness. If we are constantly doing, it's hard to be present. In yoga, for example, we rest in child's pose, mountain pose, or *shavasana* (corpse pose) as ways to honor the practice of being still. These postures require just as much effort as those that move and flow or demand engaged muscles. Stillness is pure. Stillness has no intention but to be in the moment.

If you are overwhelmed with projects and tasks, remember to invite stillness into the practice of cleansing. Sometimes, we focus so much on getting a practice "right," we overdo out of obligation or perfectionism, and we miss the lesson when we set something down.

If your cleansing routine has been all about doing, try not doing. Sit for a few quiet minutes at the start of your day. Don't turn on your phone or TV. Sip coffee or tea. Observe the moment. It's okay not to dive into journaling, yoga, or meditation. It's helpful to let our body settle after sleep and before getting up and continuing through our day for the same reasons it's necessary to practice shavasana at the end of a yoga class. It's okay, and a benefit, to be still. Not every cleansing ritual requires doing. Not every yoga pose requires effort. Check in with the moments you are still, and know they are all still part of the practice.

DAY 23

An anxious mind is easy to feed. When we get stuck on something, the anxiety about being stuck makes everything worse. Even though our reaction may be to do more, feeling stuck is asking us to slow down, to be still for a moment until we know what to do next. It's a lot harder to hear our intuition when we are worried or in a state of panic. If there is something particularly confusing or anxiety producing, try sitting for a moment and observe the sensations in your body. What does confusion feel like? Where do you sense anxiety or tightness? If the urge to jump up and "act" is strong, take a few breaths. Watch the inhale and exhale through the nostrils. Be patient, and let your body and your nervous system settle.

When anxious, the mind is especially active, racing with stories and narratives. Fear will continue to force us into impulsive decision-making as long as we let it rule our thoughts and our cells, as long as we continue to feed the stories in our mind. The body speaks to us in sensations, not stories or narratives. When we offer the body space to breathe, truth arrives in the form of deep knowing. Breathing through anxiety and practicing stillness over action is an excellent way to engage in saucha. The mind is full of stories and distraction, and when we create space through stillness, when we cleanse the body and the moment with a few breaths, we are better able to hear. Only then, from a place of calm and ease, should you act.

DAY 24
Dirgha

Dirgha pranayama is a three-part yogic breath. Dirgha opens space in the body to receive a full inhale and complete a full exhale. We create space for dirgha by sitting tall, lengthening the spine, and observing the natural path of the breath.

Begin seated, lying down, or standing. Place your hands on your belly and notice the breath. When you inhale, the belly expands, and when you exhale, the belly contracts. Notice this. Next, move your hands up to your rib cage. When you inhale, the breath first expands the belly and then moves into the lungs. The rib cage flares out and fills with breath. The exhale takes the same route—first contracting the rib cage and then the belly. The final and third part of dirgha is to rest the hands on the collarbones. On the inhale, the belly will expand, then the ribs, and finally, the collarbones will lift.

When you're paying attention, you'll notice all three parts. On the exhale, the collarbones will drop, the rib cage will contract, and the belly will deflate. Dirgha pranayama has many benefits. Not only does this practice encourage full inhales and exhales, cleansing our cells and our organs, but it also settles the mind and allows for inward focus. Dirgha is a useful technique when we feel anxious or too much in our head. Just a few minutes of practicing the three-part breath will open space, move energy, and shift your perspective to a clearer view.

DAY 25

Good or bad, joyful or tragic, easy or challenging—life will always bring new experiences and new sensations. There is a guarantee in all of existence, and that guarantee is change. Everything is temporary. We live, age, and die. Childhood is temporary. So are jobs and relationships. Even the ones that last will change, grow, and adjust with new circumstances and new perspectives. Being aware of the temporality of all things can help us to appreciate the good and accept the bad.

As human beings, we change through our experiences. Often, a very challenging experience points us to exactly what we are meant to learn. Challenging experiences bring us in touch with this undeniable center, referred to by author and psychologist Stephen Cope as "the still point … a pulsing, living stream of energy, of light, emerging from the source that is beyond time, beyond place, beyond personality."[1] Within us is a center and a truth that always exists. During particularly challenging times, and through yoga, we can access the still point. We can breathe fully into the belly. We can engage the core during a balance pose. We can sit in stillness and place a hand on our own heart. When we accept the temporality of life and circumstance, we are able to stay with the current moment because we know it won't always be this way. We can be patient and abiding through chaos, injury, or setback because we are assured it will change. We can also find strength and solace in knowing *we* are still in there. Our indestructible center remains despite outside circumstance.

....

1. Cope, *Yoga and the Quest for the True Self*, 152.

DAY 26

Part of cleansing through yoga is removing layers of false Self in order to access our truth. Sometimes, as life happens, we allow a person or situation to affect our sense of who we are. When we are betrayed, hurt, abused, or taken advantage of, false beliefs about our worthiness and what we deserve bubble to the surface, and we might want to shoulder all the blame.

There is a part of us that defies any circumstance. And that is our true Self, our essence, and our center. Our essence is the part of us beneath every single layer—beneath our age, our experiences, our labels, and our circumstance. Our center is indestructible. The truth of who we are is unbreakable and unchanging. This is the part of us that cannot be affected by other people, supposed failures, challenges, or tragedies. Of course we are affected when life doesn't go our way or when we experience loss. But it's important to remember that these experiences need not define who we are. Not getting the job may mean someone else was better qualified, but has little to do with our capacity. Being betrayed by someone we trust does not mean we are undeserving of love, but may reveal the other person's weaknesses.

Our experiences and our reactions to them point to core beliefs about ourselves that may or may not be true. Even terrible occurrences can be catalysts for healing if we view them as an opportunity to go within. Remember to seek inquiry rather than answers. How does this situation make you question yourself? What is being awakened in you, and is that story true today? Like rain cleanses the earth and allows for new growth, so, too, can whatever situation you are facing.

DAY 27

Often, our practice begins with vigor and excitement. But after a bit, our willingness fades. We wonder if it is working. We become bored or indifferent. We forget why we were doing something in the first place. During any meaningful practice, we come up against doubt and resistance. The hardest times to come down to my mat are the days I don't want to. Sometimes, I force myself. I either have a terrible practice, or I am pulled out of my funk. I do believe that when we at least show up, we are made better.

Other times, I recognize that today might not be the day for a physical practice. Today, I might need to breathe for five minutes. Today, I might need to drink more water and take a nap.

When we are in the practice of saucha, cleansing and purity, we begin to see yoga everywhere. Yoga becomes more than an order of postures on a mat. Yoga becomes heart centered, which means we honor ourselves as we are.

This doesn't mean we should give up at the first sign of resistance or setback. All hope is not lost. Recall your intention and why you are here. Acknowledge small or big shifts that have already manifested in your life. Trust that this process is working. In the end, yoga aims to bring us to peace and contentment. We are not at peace when we are solely pushing forward at all costs in order to reach a goal. We are also not content when we stop showing up for ourselves. When resistance arrives, welcome it in, and make the choice that is best for you.

DAY 28

"Hey, that's interesting." I say this to myself sometimes. When something unusual or uncomfortable arrives in my psyche, I invite my witness to take over, and I say from a point of neutrality, *"Hey, that's interesting."* Interesting stuff arrives all the time when we practice yoga. We might feel the need to label these "interesting" sensations as grief, sadness, anger, trauma, joy, fear, or love. But when we enact the witness, we don't need to name anything.

Often, simply by noticing the sensation, something already starts to heal. We don't always need to figure everything out. Just like our anatomical body functions whether we know it or not, our emotional body does the same. Sensations are energy, and like all energy, they move. While it is important to acknowledge what might be behind the sensation, it can be equally powerful to observe the sensation building, cresting, and dissipating. Not every emotion points to the story we are telling ourselves. From a somatic perspective, sensations that arrive in the body don't need to be analyzed in order to heal. They only need to be watched lovingly, kindly, and without judgment. This is why yoga heals without us needing to know what's happening. We feel lighter after our practice because the body is smart, and it has released unwanted emotions because we have stayed with them and given them space to move.

DAY 29

As we near the end of our practice of cleansing, notice what has opened up in your body, your home, and your being. Surely there are still projects you haven't gotten to. Maybe you are in the churning stage, and everything feels messier than when you began. Cleaning out is messy because we have let it build up. Life is busy, and it's easier to shove something away in a drawer instead of finding a better place for it, especially when we are rushed. When guests are arriving or I am cleaning house, I am very guilty of getting clutter out of sight quickly rather than actually dealing with it.

After years of surviving life's responsibilities and busyness, it's likely you had little time to focus on yourself. When there is a lot to get done, self-care practices are the first to go. *I'll tend to myself later—when life has calmed down.*

It's hard to notice when life actually catches up to you. We rarely see that it's time to start honoring ourselves until we have gotten sick, had a real mess, or are a frazzled wreck. Author and expert on yoga's ethical practices Deborah Adele describes this unpresence as "living on the leftovers of where we have been or the preparations of where we are going."[2] In practicing saucha, you have recognized the importance of presence, of tending to the moment, little by little. No matter what happened so far or how you applied the theme of saucha, don't be hard on yourself. Recognize the small practices and the new insights gained. Purity exists in this moment, and there is no rush.

....
2. Adele, *The Yamas & Niyamas*, 113.

DAY 30

Thoughts are powerful. Thoughts run our mind and then shape our experience. When we attach stories to these thoughts, we create positive or negative experiences in our lives. We've all done this. We have all seen firsthand how a bad attitude toward something can ruin what might have been an okay situation. Not only does saucha teach us the purity in the present moment, but it begs us to remain here, still and inquisitive, in order to avoid clinging to the past or worrying about the future.

Saucha teaches us truth beyond the muddying of our critical thoughts and the distraction of our story. Earlier, you wrote down an intention. Rather than running full force toward it, you have learned an amount of trust and letting go. Your intention is set, and that is enough. Now is the time to be still, intimate with the present moment as if it were a long-lost love. Free from clutter in our environment, and free from heaviness in our soul, we can take full breaths. We can actually notice the breath and the spaces it fills. We can roll out our mat in the cleared-out room and practice. Our mind is less foggy, and we make decisions more easily.

Our intention guides us and holds us on our path. As long as we continue toward our intention, we don't need to worry about detours or slow progress. Our hearts are full, open, and curious. We have made space, and now, we can welcome it all in.

PRACTICE 2
The Body

Yoga is a physical practice. Asana (the postures) provides benefits for the body and also the mind. As a result of your practice, your body may change—muscles may tone and strengthen, flexibility can increase, balance can improve. You may feel better equipped for other physical activity, such as walking, running, or doing chores. You may sleep better. Yoga postures tend to the body, so we experience fewer aches and pain. Yoga also improves the function of the immune system, digestion, and heart rate. After a regular yoga practice, people notice all kinds of changes and benefits, which are up to the individual to feel and notice.

Maybe more important than the physical benefits of yoga, asana can also bring a powerful shift in how we view and treat our body, which may offer surprising benefits we hadn't considered. Yoga offers kindness and compassion to a tired body, a body exhausted from all the negative self-talk and striving. After a lifetime of disassociating from the body, and regarding it as something to criticize, it can be eye-opening to realize the body is actually a friend, a wise teacher, and an ally, rather than something separate to rail against.

DAY 31

What does it mean to befriend the body? Yes, it means to eat well, stop criticizing, and accept yourself as you are. But in yoga, befriending the body means so much more. Even if someone has a healthy relationship with body image and food, most of us have never really been taught how to interact with our body as a resource and as a voice we can trust. In fact, we've probably been conditioned to not trust our body or our intuition. We've probably been taught to rely on others, on outside appearance and opinion, or on societal and cultural norms for validation, especially when it comes to the body.

Your body is not only a friend but a trusted ally. Your body knows every secret, every sting, and every heartfelt experience you've been through. And your body keeps these experiences tucked inside cells and muscles, throbbing, pulsing, and living, even if your mind remains unaware.

In yoga, befriending the body means accepting all its parts, forming a healthy relationship, and treating the body you were given with love and compassion. It also means noticing sensations, listening when something arrives, and learning to trust your intuition. Befriending the body means slowly undoing most—if not all—of what we have been taught when it comes to body awareness and learning how to listen, how to trust, and how to compassionately heal from the illusion that our body is against us.

DAY 32

I did yoga for more than twenty-five years before I understood it as a compassionate practice and not exercise. While my yoga practice was healthy for my body, my motives were a bit skewed.

I attended a yoga class several months after having my first baby. My body had changed as a result of pregnancy and lack of exercise, and I wanted to get back to my "old self." So, I sat in lotus pose silently judging my body. I glared at my stomach, which I called bloated and unattractive. I compared my entire form to another body in the room. I regretted the T-shirt I had thrown on and wished I would have combed my hair. I decided to go on a diet immediately when I got home.

How many times have you attended a yoga class or other self-care activity only to compare yourself to others and, as a result, feel worse afterward than when you arrived? According to Stephen Cope, "When we're judging or criticizing our experience, we cannot be fully in it."[3] I notice myself judging and comparing not just during yoga but in my parenting, my relationships, and my job. Yoga is meant to bring us into our experience, and the body is a great teacher. You may start to notice when the critical voice arrives, in a pose or during your day, and how berating it can be regarding your body and your abilities. When the critical voice gets loud, gently ask yourself if it is serving you in the moment. If not, bring your attention back to something in the present and know that any criticism or judgment is unproductive.

. . . .

3. Cope, *Yoga and the Quest for the True Self*, 186.

DAY 33

When I was going through my divorce, I was in so much pain, so much grief, and so much unknown that I fought to avoid the feelings. The intensity of my emotions only subsided when I fell asleep at night, and when I woke in the morning, I didn't know how to face another day of such acute sensation. To cope, I stayed focused on the good that would come out of my hardship. Maybe I would be happier; maybe my kids would be happier; maybe I could learn and grow from my past. Maybe … I could heal. Maybe … I could love again.

I tried to build myself up through exercise and self-improvement. I redecorated the house. I got a new job. I shifted everything on the outside to reflect the life I wanted.

Not all bad. But what I didn't do was stay with the current pain. I didn't hold myself inside the heartache and sadness. I didn't sit with my emotions and allow them to consume my body. I thought maybe if I was strong enough, optimistic enough, and faithful enough I could bypass the discomfort of the grieving process and simply skip over to self-actualization.

The body knows when something is being ignored. Anything unprocessed in the body will resurface until it is healed. It's okay to stay busy after loss, but allow time to sit with yourself as well. I've learned that difficult and even painful emotions won't kill us. Sometimes, the best thing we can do for our bodies is to listen to what they are telling us.

DAY 34

I often have students stand in mountain pose, place one hand on their belly, and one on their heart. We begin a class this way or arrive here after a few invigorating postures. With a hand on our belly and a hand on our heart, we can feel. In feeling, we can observe. In observing, we can pinpoint sensation. What does your heartbeat feel like? What is the sensation of the breath entering and leaving? Where are your feet? What is the sensation of the surface beneath them?

Tuning in to the body through sensations brings an observer's mind to our practice. As an observer, we are neutral. Sensations are felt and noticed but not labeled. We witness the body as it is—without attaching a reason or a story. The only purpose becomes the act of noticing. The mind is an elaborate storyteller. Naturally, and often without realizing it, we attach stories and write narratives around any thought that arrives. Through yoga and cultivating the witness, we can train the mind to simply observe. When the mind becomes a witness, we are free from stories, past experience, and false narrative. We are wholly present and attuned to what is happening in the body. As researcher Bessel van der Kolk writes, "One of the clearest lessons from contemporary neuroscience is that our sense of ourselves is anchored in a vital connection with our bodies."[4] By observing sensations, we are able to more clearly observe ourselves. Sensations become a way to stop the active mind and a way to access deeper levels of awareness and a more real sense of who we are.

. . . .
4. van der Kolk, *The Body Keeps the Score*, 274.

DAY 35

Kripalu Center for Yoga and Health, where I completed my teacher training, is named after Swami Kripalu, a speaker, teacher, and yogi who arrived in the United States from India in 1977 and inspired thousands of people on their spiritual path. *Kripalu* means "compassion." So, when people ask me what type of yoga I practice, I say, "compassionate yoga."

On the mat, compassionate yoga looks like taking care of my body and my needs. It looks like taking rest and not trying to force an impressive pose for the sake of my ego. It also looks like pushing myself, when I know I can, to my edge in order to try something new. It looks like allowing myself to be challenged in order to remember what I am capable of.

Compassionate yoga looks like all the lessons I need to learn and practice in life. Compassionate yoga yields so much curiosity and self-observation. I remember lessons from my yoga practice and try them out in other situations. I add rest during a particularly busy day. I make time for play, fun, and smiling. I laugh at myself when I fall. I try hard things. I listen to my heart when it speaks to me. I sit still and breathe when I don't know what to do next.

When we embody compassion as a core principle in our life, we intuitively make different decisions. We choose to be kind to ourselves and others. There are not as many mistakes made, a lot less injury and hurt feelings, and a lot more love and tenderness to go around.

DAY 36

Enacting the witness and practicing compassion for ourselves and our body goes much deeper than treating ourselves with kindness. According to Swami Kripalu, "The highest form of spiritual practice is self-observation without judgment."[5] The first time I heard these words, my mind was blown wide open, and I almost couldn't grasp their meaning. *Observe myself without judgment? This is a spiritual practice?*

As I meditated on the depth of this practice, I began to feel hopeful. What would it look like to let go of all judgment and critique? What would it feel like to practice a pose or a life situation without the qualities of proving, perfectionism, or blame? If self-observation without judgment is a spiritual practice, how will the results not only affect me but ripple out to others and the world?

I'll admit, learning to observe without judgment seems impossible at first. Accepting unflattering parts of ourselves, such as anger, jealousy, or impatience, feels like condoning and like we will never change. Actually, when we observe ourselves without judgment, we welcome in more insight, more truths, and more opportunity for change. We also learn how to observe others with the same understanding and grace. As we uncover our own pain points as a result of our experience, we become aware of other people's pain and shortcomings. The entire world becomes an opportunity to practice awareness, and suddenly, we are living compassionately always. We begin to recognize the humanness in all of us.

....

5. Kripalu, "Swami Kripalu's Inspiration for Yoga Teachers."

DAY 37

I decided to challenge myself and complete 108 sun salutations in honor of the winter solstice, my gesture to the Universe, my readiness for death and rebirth. I attended a yoga class on the shortest day of the year, anxious to say I did it. The instructor placed ten buttons in a vertical line in front of our mats and told us to move one button for every ten salutations as a way to keep track.

"This is not about completing 108 sun salutations," began the instructor. "This is about endurance, honor, and being present."

I felt I had missed something. I was hyperfocused on the end goal—I could already visualize all ten buttons on the opposite side of my mat, symbolizing victory.

When our time was up, three buttons remained on the right side of my mat. I had only completed seventy-eight sun salutations.

I am enough; this is enough. I said to myself.

Throughout the class, I had slowly begun to let go of the number and listen when my body needed to rest or slow down. There is no magic number. There is no magic pose. The point of completing 108 sun salutations is not to knock out the physical practice with no regard for the body. When the body senses we are honoring it, we experience contentment and love, which we would not know if we had just bulldozed ahead. Even though I didn't complete the 108 sun salutations, I benefited greatly from the practice. I learned to let go of the number and my desire for achievement—or at least the image of achievement I had in my head. I learned my body was enough—just as it is.

DAY 38

Developing a practice that offers choices for our body on the mat helps us to also honor the body in life. Every choice during yoga is an opportunity to respect the body rather than regard it as something to be dismissed or ignored. My eating disorder has been a great teacher for the ways I silenced my body and my inner voice. While active in my addiction, pangs of hunger were never acknowledged with food or nourishment. Constantly dismissed, my body eventually became accustomed to feeling hungry as a way of existence. My body also learned that pleas would not be answered, so my intuition and inner knowing got shoved down right along with the cravings for food. At my core, I trained myself not to matter. Just like I refused to nourish my body with regular meals, I also refused to acknowledge my emotions, my hurts, and my desires. Pleasurable experiences brought guilt and shame. When I did enjoy food, I immediately threw it up afterward. Yoga gave me the opportunity to practice loving my body through poses, through observation, and through choices. I started listening to my body, and this act of self-love felt so much better than dismissing it.

Maybe your issue is not an eating disorder. Maybe there are other ways you practice self-refusal, such as not sleeping, overcommitting, or overworking. Maybe your body has learned to compensate by no longer making itself known. During your yoga practice, make a choice that honors what your body is asking for and see what arrives. Trust may arrive. Love may arrive. And you may realize how kind and loving it feels to acknowledge the body.

DAY 39

For thousands of years, yogis have understood a connection between the physical body and the subtle body, which is the deeper layers of Self, the emotional set point, and the place where experience is stored. Ancient yogis knew their physical practice benefited the body but also that it brought other transformative experiences, such as greater self-awareness and heightened intuition. Today, psychology and neuroscience prove what the yogis discovered long ago: that every experience, every heartache, and every tragedy is not only experienced by our mind but also by our body.[6] This knowledge helps us better understand how yoga is an effective practice in healing our entire being.

The nervous system regulates every single autonomic function—the heartbeat, the immune system, breath, digestion, and so on. When the nervous system is off-balance, whether from acute trauma or prolonged stress, our bodies respond.[7] We are agitated, we get sick, and we can't think. Most of us are probably living in a heightened state of stress on a regular basis, which leaves little room for self-actualization or fulfillment. Poses and breath regulate the nervous system as well as the emotional Self. At minimum, yoga balances the nervous system and welcomes in calm. But on a deeper level, yoga grants access to our greatest potential by forming a relationship with our inner Self, which has the power to heal, transform, and release us from much of our suffering.

....

6. van der Kolk, *The Body Keeps the Score*, 274–75.

7. van der Kolk, *The Body Keeps the Score*, 269.

DAY 40
Shavasana (Corpse Pose)

Lie down on your back, and let your feet splay open to the sides. Feel the flesh of your calves roll onto the outer edges. Let your thighs be apart. Notice the surface beneath your shoulder blades and how the bones feel against it. Observe the back of your head and the point where it makes contact with the surface. Rest your arms along your sides, palms face up. Close your eyes. Watch the breath. Keep your inner gaze pinned to the awareness of breath just as it is— the inhale and exhale.

If you've ever been to a yoga class, you've probably ended in shavasana. Shavasana is the final resting pose after the physical practice. Shavasana symbolizes completion. The practice has ended. Shavasana also symbolizes death and a rebirth when we emerge. After our yoga practice, we realize something has changed. Something has shifted. At a cellular level, whether we know it or not, we are not the same.

Despite the minimal physical effort it takes to lie down, eyes closed, body unmoving, shavasana has never been an easy pose for me. I squirm and I fidget. I anticipate when we will be allowed to come out. My mind is already wandering ahead to the next thing. Many yogis experience this. Some even feel anxious while attempting to be so still. It has helped me to let go of my fear that there is a wrong way. Shavasana is a reset, not a conquest. The best I can offer myself on any day is a compassionate look at what might be going on.

Here's something else that may shock you (it did in my rule-bound mind). Shavasana can be done *anytime*. Not just at the end of yoga class.

DAY 41

I spent a lot of my life navigating people and situations, trying to figure out who to show up as and which mask to wear. I learned what people wanted, what they needed from me, and I skillfully became that. The problem, other than the entire charade being exhausting, was that I never understood who I was, what I needed, or what made me happy. I also hid parts of myself I was ashamed of. I hid some for the sake of societal expectations and some because I felt they were just too dark to share.

Yoga grants us permission. Yoga asks us to bring our whole Self to the mat, whether it's light, dark, happy, sad, optimistic, or bewildered. Yoga implores that we make the appropriate choices for our body in that moment, whether it is to flow, to stay, to reach, or to rest. I didn't know I had the power or the permission to complete myself by accepting all the parts—my harsh edges *and* my soft center.

To my amazement, when we show up as our whole Self, life gets a lot easier. Instead of trying to win people over who aren't good for us anyway, we let them naturally drift away. Instead of holding resentment, we feel content. I learned that the greatest, purest validation doesn't come from others but from myself.

DAY 42

Yoga is called a path because a regular practice takes you to a different place from where you began. I call yoga a return because our practice gives back to us all the parts we have abandoned. These are the parts we have been ashamed to show up as. They're the parts that crave our attention.

Teaching yoga online has taught me a lot about what showing up really looks like. My students and clients have shown me what true bravery is. They show up tired. They show up between job shifts. They show up amid chaos with children and pets vying for their attention just behind the door. They show up unsure, embarrassed, and afraid. They show up wondering if they really have time for yoga today or if any of it really matters. Yet they show up.

Your yoga practice doesn't care if you're angry, lost, or heartbroken. Your yoga practice doesn't care if the house is messy or the dog is barking. Bring it. Bring everything you are to your mat. Bring your tears, your screams, and your sighs. Surrender your body to the breath and the postures. Allow yourself to be who you are without expectation or the need to dim your emotions. Bring your whole Self to your practice, and see what that looks like. Give it a try. It's interesting what we hold on to, and we may not ever realize the heaviness it creates until we give ourselves permission to let it flow.

DAY 43

The word *integration* gets thrown around a lot in yoga—and for good reason. But I always wondered what this word meant in terms of yoga and the body. What are we integrating? Why is integration so important?

Most simply, to integrate an experience is to feel it. Yoga offers space to feel emotions and physical sensations, thus integrating anything, from that morning to past events. Everyday events can be integrated quickly. The event happens, the body becomes alarmed, and when it ends, we move on. However, more intense experience can take longer to integrate. To demonstrate the importance of integration, David A. Treleaven offers a personalized approach to recognizing trauma or dis-integration. Rather than define trauma according to the event, he suggests "looking at one's individual response—specifically whether or not they could integrate the experience."[8]

If we don't integrate our experience, an event becomes traumatic. Our body reacts to life in a way that is disconnected from our senses and our true experience. The brain might shut down these experiences, and we can't be free. If you are in the midst of something painful, move gently. Begin by noticing sensations in your body. Become aware of your body as an ally here to help and teach you. Remind yourself: *I am safe*. Stay open when uncomfortable emotions arrive, and always stop when you need to. Feeling your experience as sensation helps to integrate.

....
8. Treleaven, *Trauma-Sensitive Mindfulness*, 13.

DAY 44

I was in a writing class, and the assignment was to explain a benefit of our book for readers. I wrote, "Yoga can help us feel less lonely." My partner responded, "Really? How does yoga help with loneliness?"

Yoga helps us stay with difficult emotions, therefore allowing them to move and pass through. It is natural for human beings to shut down around feelings. We're unable to understand them and afraid to become overwhelmed. We close our heart, literally and emotionally. Our shoulders cave inward. We build armor and remain disconnected from people and activities. We can feel lonely while in a room full of people and enjoy a sense of deep connection while in solitude. Emotions are complex sensations. We can feel opposing emotions, at once excited and afraid, sad and relieved, lonely and safe.

Through regular practice, we can get better at staying with opposing sensations. Our feelings don't always match logic or our surroundings, yet they are all valid and meant to be felt. Yoga helps us feel less lonely because we get comfortable in our own skin. We become aware and accepting of our emotions. While our protection instinct might be to remain guarded and closed, we trust in the process of slowly allowing ourselves to peel open—of allowing our real emotions to flow. We develop ways to honor ourselves and, therefore, love ourselves. We don't feel alone because even when we are with ourselves, on our mat or in a meditation, we sense connection. We sense purpose. We sense that we are never actually alone.

DAY 45
Goddess Pose

Stand with legs wide apart, feet turned open. Press your palms together at heart center. Take an inhale. Exhale and slowly bend your knees. Come down as low as you can into a wide-legged squat, keeping the knees open and pulling back. Find your edge. Find the essential place where you sense effort but not strain. Stay. Observe as the sensations build. Muscles wake up. Thighs tingle and shake. Stay. A slow burn ignites. Stay. Doubt arrives. Stay. For one more breath (or two), stay.

We are constantly meeting edges in life. Yoga teaches us that the edge, the point of discomfort, unsureness, or fear, is an opportunity to question everything we have thought to be true. We sustain a pose in order to observe what happens at the edge. How do we respond? What does our mind tell us? At an edge, do we stay? Do we stay in the discomfort? Can we be with the experience that the edge provides?

The accomplishment is not about how long we hold the pose. It's the self-discovery that happens along the way. To meet an edge is to be aware of our discomfort and aware of the fact that we don't know what's on the other side. When you stay for one more breath, when you question the mind that is saying you can't, when you trust that your body will not die from holding a pose, you arrive at a new place of awareness.

Maybe you are stronger than you think. Maybe you don't have to believe in the self-doubt. Maybe the voice in your head is not always accurate. Maybe your body is the wise teacher.

DAY 46

I hovered a foot or so above the ground in *phalakasana* (plank pose). With my arms straight, shoulders lined up over my wrists, and legs extended long behind me, I lowered my hips so they were even with my spine. One long, straight, excruciating line.

I shook. My core tightened, let go, and then tightened again. I imagined my abdominal muscles being sewn up with thread, which would narrow the three-finger-sized space that had formed after two pregnancies. It was as if my body, my soul, and my sanity depended on this pose.

Around this time, my life was falling apart. I was newly sober and determined in my recovery but still unsure and shaky. Nothing was natural. Every decision was deliberate—run through a rational checklist and set of suggested tools. *If you go to a party and there's alcohol, make sure you have a way out. Have nonalcoholic options on hand. If you think about drinking, call a supportive friend or your sponsor. Like a wild bunny that wriggles off fear and quietly hops away, let yourself breathe and shake, and the craving will pass.*

Plank pose has taught me so much about my body, my mind, and life itself. Plank pose has taught me that my body can change, which means I can change. Plank pose has, in fact, brought the gap in my abdominals back together, which I thought was impossible after having children. Yoga is a practice that honors the comeback. If you're weak, yoga helps you stay strong. If you're confused, yoga brings clarity. If you're lost, yoga leads you back to yourself.

DAY 47

My ten-year-old year old said to me after an argument, "When you're inside your emotions, it's hard to think straight." Such insight from my young son.

When we get overcome with emotion, it can result in unhealthy habits or destructive actions. The problem lies not in the emotions themselves but in the mind's attachment to them. In yoga, the ego is called the *ahamkara*, the I-maker. The I-maker gives us our identity and is a necessary aspect of being human. We form an identity through likes and dislikes, interests, and passions. The problem arrives when we overidentify with the I-maker. We forget that we are actually none of these ego-driven things. It is very easy for the ego to become wound up in thoughts, especially when there is strong or negative emotion present. A thought arrives, and we swiftly get pulled away by the emotion. The mind adds a story, and we are swept further into illusion.

In a heightened emotional state, with our ego running wild, it's hard to think straight. So, what can we do? How do we achieve a helpful awareness of ego? It's possible to observe thoughts without attaching to a story. Take a few minutes to be still. Observe thoughts that come in, and notice how they change. Notice where your mind wanders as a result of the thought. If you don't attach to the wandering mind, what happens to the thought? We are able to control the ahamkara when we understand that our thoughts are not who we are. By having discernment to disengage from the story, we make healthier decisions, react less violently, and gain a better understanding of our true Self.

DAY 48

In a world with so much going on—personally, in our homelife, in our work life, and in larger society—it's easy to forget ourselves. It's easy to allow our body and our mental state to be pulled in all directions, wavering, tipping, flailing. We have much to give, but without a strong sense of Self, we can't be of help to anyone.

Just as our center keeps us in alignment on the mat, our personal truth and integrity need to remain intact during our day-to-day. In a balance pose, the best way to stay upright is not to fight the pose and strain but to engage the core, lengthen, and stand a little taller. In life, we must also move and breathe from this centered, knowing space with calmness rather than desperation.

The more we practice, the stronger we get. Poses become easier. Balance becomes attainable. Our emotional state is the same way. The more we practice honoring ourselves and standing tall, the easier life gets. No longer are we guilted into staying when our gut tells us to leave. No longer are we overextended when we know we need to back off. No longer are we silent when we have the words to say.

Before any big decision or when the world appears to swirl and crest around you, you can return to your center just like we do in yoga. You can pause, be still, and guide your awareness inward. Let go of fighting the outside circumstance and stay focused on your inner knowing. It is from this place of centered strength that we can be most effective in the world.

DAY 49

Before any physical movement, begin each practice in stillness. Arrive seated in a chair or on your cushion. Invite internal focus by closing your eyes. Become aware of an inner world, one that needs attention. Breathe. Watch the breath as if for the first time. The breath is happening now, so it will anchor you in the present.

The centering at the beginning of practice tells our body and our nervous system to calm down, to settle in, and to shift the gaze inside. Only after several minutes of stillness and breath do we begin to move. Slowly, we bend our spine. Mindfully, we stretch our limbs. With care and attention, we witness our body and all its sensations. The body is an entire world of sensation. Tight muscles, air on skin, physical aches. We might also notice emotional tenderness, waves of grief or joy, heaviness around the ribs, agitation in the throat, or dampness behind the eyes.

As we hold our gaze on these sensations, we also observe their impermanence. We've all heard the cliché of "This too shall pass." A mindful yoga practice allows us to experience this truth firsthand. Sensations change. They might not disappear, but they change. Everything is impermanent—states of joy and states of pain. When we are able to notice the subtle shifts of sensation and the inevitable nature of impermanence, we are better able to stay rather than run. We can accept where we are and be present because we know *this too shall pass*.

DAY 50

You are building a foundation. By making space and tuning in to the body, you are accomplishing more than you know. It may seem simple to notice one breath at a time, to bring the body into a pose and observe, but the effects of this new way of experiencing reach deep into your cells and penetrate the interior layers of Self. Buried wounds and tucked-away experience begin to reveal themselves. When we observe sensations in the body, the inner world is illuminated and brought to the surface. The power of this awareness is that we travel deeper inward and know there is still more—an even deeper knowing we can access. Yogis believed the layers of Self to be infinite.[9] The inward journey is one of continual cleansing, uncovering, and bringing to light.

After some practice observing surface sensation, you might start to notice the mind letting go even more. Once focused on the felt sensation of breath, for example, the mind might open to an exploration of pure awareness. This experience can feel like a trance, as if you have lost track of time. Trance states may happen during yoga or during any activity where the subconscious is awakened, such as writing, cooking, or gardening. We are not operating according to rational thought but through a sense of deeper knowing. There is a force other than "us" guiding our activity. Do not be alarmed by or fearful toward these states of awareness. Your practice is working! We often come out of these moments with a sense of peace or longing. We crave more and want to return to them. We want to remember those parts of ourselves because it feels like home.

....
9. Cope, *The Wisdom of Yoga*, 84.

DAY 51
Standing Balance Pose

Stand on one leg, and raise the other in front of you with a bent knee. Let the lifted foot be soft, dangling off the ankle. Lift the arms out to the sides with elbows slightly bent and hands also soft, hanging off the wrists. Press into the entire foot of the standing leg, and lengthen through the crown of your head. Allow your standing foot to ground you as the lifted leg and arms are free to hang.

In a standing balance pose, notice the effort as well as the softness and ease. If balance is unsteady, discover where you can engage more effort and welcome in more ease. Notice where effort is fruitless, such as in the hanging hands and foot. Tensing the muscles in the arms, for example, brings no increased steadiness to the posture. Squeezing the hands into fists or clenching the jaw does not improve balance. You must find more surface beneath the sole of the standing foot. You must pull up on the thigh and engage the core, so the pelvis tilts into alignment. Guide the shoulders down and elongate the neck. Feel the tops of your ears floating upward and let the teeth separate.

In balance, explore how you might find more comfort and steadiness. What are you holding that is unneeded? What are you ignoring that would make a difference? Asana is not about striking a pose and holding on for dear life. Asana encourages subtle shifts in our energy, so the pose becomes equal parts ease and effort. Find a place that is comfortable but still requires focus.

DAY 52

How many times have you done something, made a quick decision, only to regret it later? How many times have you had to backtrack to make up for something you wish you hadn't done? It's easy to react rather than be still. We feel we have to act right away because what we are actually interested in is not the decision but the belief that by acting, we will alleviate our pain.

Stillness before action will bring clarity. And we are less likely to do something we regret. When you sit still and let a choice wash over you, when you imagine your choice and feel it, your body often tells you if it is right. You'll be able to "feel" if you are actually at peace with your decision. We might be weighing two options, which is limited thinking. There are infinite possibilities and infinite choices to every situation. One option we rarely consider is the choice to do nothing—and wait.

Advertising plays into our fears all the time, and begs us to act without thinking. That's why we see deals and banners that claim "Don't miss out!" and "Only a few days left!" Advertising doesn't want us to sit still. Advertising wants us to pounce.

Think of your life this way. Are you taking the time to sit still, or are you pouncing? Are you trying so hard to rid yourself of pain you're behaving outside of everyone's best interests, including your own? It is only in stillness that you will be open to multiple options and multiple paths. More will always be revealed if we can just sit still.

DAY 53

If you want something to change, change something. Yoga reminds us that it's important to honor ourselves, which includes recognizing emotions and being honest when something hurts or disappoints us. But we don't need to stay too long in our discomfort. When you are in a yoga pose and something hurts, there are many ways to adjust. Take a breath, use a block, or modify the pose in some way. When we recognize discomfort in our practice, we consider our options and make an important change. Discomfort and pain in life are no different; we can acknowledge discomfort and still take action to move forward.

There is a big difference between being present and wallowing. Wallowing is hopeless and victimizing. Wallowing for too long pulls us further into a place of guilt, shame, and self-loathing where it's hard to see a way out. Of course you can give yourself space to feel your feelings. You don't need to rush being present and tuned in to where you are. But there should be a kind and loving intention behind the acknowledgment of yourself. There should also be an awareness of your greatness; you might feel sad or lost right now, but you know you are capable of more than you think. You know you are strong. You know this painful spot might motivate you to take brave action.

Unlike wallowing, which makes us feel helpless, a healthy acknowledgment of emotions allows us to feel empowered. If we want something to change, we don't need to assume we have no control. We can change one small thing, be it a habit, an interaction, our schedule, or our environment. Our discomfort shows us where to adjust.

DAY 54

Ever notice how you look different in photos than you imagine your-self to look? Our reflection is distorted because we can't see ourselves outside of ourselves. Our entire experience happens within the body and the mind. Even others don't see a true version. Their perception of us is based on their own experience, their own ego, and their own mind. According to the Yoga Sutras, "the Self will always be falsely represented by the ego until ignorance is removed."[10]

Everything we tell ourselves about who we are is probably not true. The true Self—the original Self—is not based on experience or perception. The true Self is not muddied or manipulated by ego. Yoga seeks to remove ego and therefore remove illusion. Yoga seeks to illuminate the original soul and bring truth into light.

Anything the ego tells us, whether grand or inferior, about our-selves or someone else is a reflection of our experience and therefore not necessarily accurate. Once we start to understand the ego as a lens, a mirror, we can pause before quick reaction. We get better at questioning the mind in order to discern truth from illusion. Are we acting in accordance with our true Self or as a reflection of our expe-rience? This is a long and patient process. We must make progress and then regress. We never give up on our practice because inside our practice, the true Self enters. Without ego, we are free from percep-tion, labels, and who we believe ourselves to be. We glimpse less of the ego during practice so we can behave with less of the ego in life.

....
10. Satchidananda, *The Yoga Sutras of Patanjali*, 84.

DAY 55

My dad taught me to write a pro/con list whenever I had a difficult decision to make. He said a list makes the answer clear and takes your emotions out of it. So, when weighing my options to get divorced, I wrote a list. No offense to my dad but, for my divorce, a pro/con list was not helpful. Everything about my divorce showed up as a con. All I saw staring at me were catastrophic cons: a broken family, traumatized children, loneliness, financial ruin, disapproval from God and all of society.

Then, in the "pro" column I wrote one little phrase: "my heart."

It turns out honoring who you are and answering your own heart is the most important thing. Honoring your true Self is the winner of all lists, the ultimate deal breaker, and your ace in the hole. When you know who you are and you honor that, everything always works out.

Always? Yes, I think always. Because even if things go badly or not like you expected, you didn't abandon yourself. You didn't go against your own truth for the sake of someone else's feelings or approval. You didn't shut yourself down or make yourself small. No one is small. We are all here to take up as much space as we possibly can.

So, how do you know who you are? You listen. You start by making small choices that honor who you are, and then you practice making bigger choices. You tune in. You face how you feel rather than run or deny. You trust yourself. You love yourself. And I believe that when you love yourself, you always make the best choices.

DAY 56

Newly divorced, newly sober, and raising two boys, I practically screamed at my therapist one day, "Can someone just tell me what to do, and I'll do it, I promise."

I desperately wanted to know what to do. I firmly believed that I kept screwing up, getting it wrong, and missing the whole big point of life. *I must be missing something, or my life wouldn't look like this.*

My therapist smiled, maybe smirked, and answered, "The only one who can tell you what to do, *is you. And* you have to do the work to get there."

Darn! I wanted an easy solution. I wanted to never feel the heartbreak of an ended relationship again. I wanted to never feel the shame-filled hell that is addiction. What I didn't know how to do was trust myself. I thought my challenges were punishments. It never dawned on me they might be my path—the path into myself. No matter what your life looks like on the outside and no matter how far you are from where you thought you'd be, it is an opportunity to know yourself. You are the only one who knows yourself well enough to know the next steps. Trust that just like in a pose, the easiest, most comfortable choice may not be the best one. It's important to remember your capacity, even when you know it won't be easy, even when you don't know what will happen when you move ahead. When in doubt, stay a little longer, sustain the effort, and notice that you can.

DAY 57

Sankhya is an ancient Indian spiritual philosophy that explains two aspects of existence, *purusha* (pure consciousness) and *prakriti* (nature), which make up the entire Universe.[11] Nature includes the body, the senses, and the five elements: ether, air, fire, water, earth.

We are one with nature, formed from the same energy and subject to the same impermanence. This is why connecting with nature brings feelings of calm and peace. In nature, we are closer to the source.

In Sankhya philosophy, *manas* is the mind, one of the human elements that hides us from purusha, the soul. It's a similar idea to the ego versus the true Self. The mind keeps us tied up in stories, which place us further away from who we really are. The reason this is important to our yoga practice is because we are slowly starting to notice the difference between the mind and the observer. When we understand that the mind is a part of the body, we can observe it more objectively. Like noticing our knee tingle with sensation in a pose, we can watch the mind produce stories. We don't have to attach. Instead, we can adjust, either with a breath or a different focus.

Think about when you are in nature. You might feel like you are able to be more present. Worries and stresses seem to drift away, and you are more tuned in to what's happening right now. The body is the same way. When we are present, we can observe thoughts with less agitation. The part of us watching the thoughts is purusha—the soul, the source, and the truth.

....
11. *Kripalu Yoga Teacher Training Manual*, 2.10.

DAY 58

When we observe the body, we come to realize that a part of us—the witness—is watching the body. It is observing sensations and possibly labeling them with names or qualities. The same applies to the mind. As the witness, we watch the mind produce thoughts, feelings, and wants. The witness is able to observe both. The Sutras call the witness "the Knower or Seer. You always see your mind and body acting in front of you. You know that the mind creates thoughts; it distinguishes and desires. The Seer *knows* that but is not involved in it."[12]

In short, the Seer is able to separate itself from the body and the mind. The Seer watches all the functions and does not need to attach, and we know the Seer exists because we watch it watching. The Seer is not magical or out of reach. We do not need to overthink the Seer's purpose. We simply need to acknowledge that this part of us exists. When you begin to separate the part of you that *knows* from the part of you that *feels*, you become more in touch with your deeper Self and less affected by the natural functions and sensations of the body and the mind.

....
12. Satchidananda, *The Yoga Sutras of Patanjali*, 6.

DAY 59
Meditation in Motion

Seated or standing, come into stillness and take a few breaths. Without overthinking about what is "right" or "good," start to move your body. It might feel natural to rock or sway side to side. It might feel essential to bend forward or arch back. Your desire might be to touch each fingertip to the thumb. Continue moving freely while staying anchored to the breath until you feel the practice is complete.

A yoga practice centered in compassion teaches us that we have needs, wants, and desires and that we can honor them. We have choices about how to move next. These choices create sensation, and we can decide if we crave more sensation or less. We can decide how much to move based on the type of sensation the body is asking for.

For me, the ability to make choices for my body in the moment was foreign. I had the belief that my needs and wants were not valid or not always "correct." I wanted to get the pose right; I wanted someone else to tell me what to do and to validate my choice. It has been a powerful experience to let go of technique and honor my body during yoga. I've learned that some days my body wants high sensation or vigorous movement. I've learned that other days my body craves more stillness and ease. Knowing we have choices and the ability to make them, in yoga and in life, not only makes us responsible but also able to meet our own needs.

DAY 60

Rarely do I have someone show up to yoga who doesn't want something to change. Sure, they want the physical benefits, but they are also facing something they want out of. They come for the promise of a deep yoga experience.

What is a deep experience? What does it feel like to have a moment of pure awareness, awakening, or transformation? Is it what Richard Faulds describes as "flashes of lightning that illumine the landscape on a dark night"? Is it simple, like when Faulds quotes Swami Kripalu, who called awakening "your own experience"?[13] The Twelve Steps of Alcoholics Anonymous promises a "spiritual awakening."[14] And the Sutras call it *samyogah* (union).[15] To describe instances of my own deep experience, I would use *connection* and *truth*.

Deep yoga experience does happen. But don't ignore the smaller, less showy awakenings or expect that you will have a profound experience every single time. Yoga opens us up to these experiences in life. When you have a profound experience, such as a releasing cry or a moment of clarity, it's tempting to want this type of revelation all the time. But yoga is a discipline as well as a personal practice. If you sense you have shifted something, awakened something, or had a profound moment, then I guarantee you have, and it is the result of your own practice and inner awareness.

....

13. Faulds and Senior Teachers of Kripalu Center for Yoga & Health, *Kripalu Yoga*, 253.

14. *Alcoholics Anonymous*, 567.

15. Satchidananda, *The Yoga Sutras of Patanjali*, 107.

DAY 61

Are you in enough pain to justify healing? Have you suffered thoroughly, and who decides the tipping point? Maybe you don't need to suffer to justify healing, and maybe anyone's life is difficult enough to require some sort of recovery from being human. Your pain is valid. Just because you're not starving, homeless, or experiencing some other form of major trauma does not mean you don't have room and reason to heal. When we judge and compare our circumstance to another's in order to invalidate our own experience, we excuse ourselves from the responsibility to heal.

Our pain does not have to be monumental in order to benefit greatly from a practice of self-care and a desire to uncover wounds. Healing, like love, is available to all of us. Your unique experience matters, and the only person who needs to understand that is *you*. Simply, if you don't feel quite right, if something keeps coming up and presenting itself, you don't get to dismiss yourself. People in pain hurt other people. So, when we take time to attend to our own wounds, everyone around us benefits. I believe that when we heal ourselves, we heal the world.

Imagine a world where everyone focused on healing themselves. Imagine a world where everyone took responsibility for their own healing instead of telling others what to do. I imagine that world would be a much more compassionate, forgiving, humble, and healthy place.

PRACTICE 3
The Practice

There's a myth that yoga is simply exercise. There's a myth that yoga is about how you look in your leggings and in the pose. There's a myth that yoga is about an end goal—weight loss, flexibility, advanced postures, "mastering" something. In reality, yoga is a practice. It is something we show up for. We do our practice because we love ourselves enough to honor the parts of us that long to be acknowledged. We do our practice because, even if we can't explain it, something shifts inside every single time, and we walk away different. Maybe we were less critical of ourselves. Maybe we held a pose that once was too challenging. Over the next several readings, we will focus on what a personal yoga practice looks like, how to create one, and how to practice yoga in life. It's okay to have a goal for your practice; in fact, I encourage it. But also stay open and willing to receive new gifts, new awareness, and new possibilities in poses and in daily interactions. While you may reach a goal or a milestone, your practice never ends. Your practice is a journey into Self that affects all of those we touch. Whatever happened on the mat, that experience was ours, and now, we can share the fruits with others.

DAY 62

I've talked to many people who have tried yoga and understand the benefits but have no idea how to incorporate a consistent, mindful practice into their busy, unpredictable lives. Developing a yoga practice is not about finding enough time or the right time. It's about creating something stable that supports you no matter what life brings.

Do either of these sound like you?

+ Situation One: You like yoga. You've taken classes at a studio or online, and you feel better afterward. You promise to go more often. Then life gets in the way. Your family needs you, your job and responsibilities need you, so you put yoga off.
+ Situation Two: You like the idea of yoga, but going to a class or doing yoga on your own is overwhelming. You don't feel flexible enough or experienced enough to get started. You feel like you have a lot more to learn before you can actually *do* yoga.

If you relate to either of these scenarios, you are not alone. These are common reactions and beliefs as a result of how yoga is portrayed in Western culture. The truth is: Yoga is a personal practice that you must discover for yourself. There are no physical limitations. There is no "rule" about how often or for how long you have to practice. Yoga is not limited to classes in a studio or postures on a mat. Your yoga practice is inside you. Over the next few readings, we'll learn how to incorporate a practice into your day-to-day and how to dispel more false beliefs that may be holding you back.

DAY 63

Creating a personal yoga practice brings up a lot of resistance—not knowing poses, not having space or time, doing it wrong. Today, I am giving you the first of three suggestions for creating your own practice. The next two suggestions will be in the following two readings.

My first suggestion is to set an intention. You are welcome to go back to your intention from practice 1. Your intention can be the same, or maybe it has shifted after a few months of practice. Remember that you have already been doing yoga through cleansing, observing the body, and reading this book every day. Your daily practice is already yoga. When writing your intention, consider these questions:

+ What are you seeking with your practice?
+ What would you like to change? Is there a specific pain point or current problem you would like to be rid of?
+ List any specific goals, such as strength, balance, or clarity.

You do not need to choose only one goal. Maybe you have several things in your life you would like to change. Usually, the specifics all point to a larger aim. For example, getting stronger, making new friends, and applying for a new job all could point to a desire for more confidence. Getting more rest, having less stress, and making time for exercise all could point to a desire for slowing down.

Consider the larger aim that directs your goals. Aim your arrow by writing your intention down. Then release your intention to the Universe and know it will become reality. Your aim has set everything you desire into motion.

DAY 64

My second suggestion is to design your practice. Acknowledge your progress and create a routine that makes sense for you and your lifestyle. Have you read this book so far? Great job! Have you tried some of the poses, or do you already have a consistent yoga practice? This is progress. Decide which parts of a daily practice will realistically fit into your day. Maybe you function best in the morning, so getting up, doing the reading, and performing a bit of yoga makes sense. Maybe you are not a morning person, and it's enough just to get up and get out the door. In this case, a gentle evening practice before bed might work best for you.

Let go of any expectations of what you think a yoga practice should look like, and design something personal. Journal while you have your morning coffee and include some breath and movement afterward. Take a walk after lunch and ponder the ideas in this book. Complete a twenty-minute yoga practice before bed. Dedicate time each day, or dedicate time once a week. Commit to something manageable and then show up.

Showing up should come with some healthy resistance. If it's too easy or lackadaisical, that may be a sign that you are under-committing. You should encounter an amount of discipline when designing your practice, meaning there is effort to see it through. But don't plan something so unattainable that you will be discouraged and give up completely. Keep the following intentions in mind as you create your practice: remember, honor, love, and discipline.

DAY 65

My third suggestion is to create a sacred space. You don't need an entire room dedicated to yoga. You only need a special area that will symbolize your practice. While yoga can be done in a studio, outside, or anywhere you roll out your mat, it's nice to have a sacred space in your home that invites your practice. Lay your mat out in front of a sunny window. Light a candle in your bedroom. Declutter a corner for a chair and a bookshelf. Do something small to signify that this is a healing space—*your* space.

The more you enjoy your space, the more you will want to be in it. As we know from saucha, it's hard to observe our inner landscape when our outside surroundings are messy. Of course if you are a parent, there might be toys and clutter in your home that are inevitable. Pets, children, partners, and family members all contribute to a home full of energy and love. Your space does not have to be spotless, silent, or perfect. Just enough room to place your mat so you may arrive. Consider all the senses when creating your space. In addition to something visual, use touch, sound, taste, and smell. Have blankets and props nearby. Personalize your space. Consider meaningful objects and images. Have fun creating the sacred space that will bring much healing, insight, and growth. Your space symbolizes your readiness and your commitment.

DAY 66

Practice is a discipline, one that is continuous and takes place over a long time. We want immediate results, but the fruits of a consistent practice reveal more benefits than showing up off and on, sporadically, or only when we feel like it. Of course there will be days when we need to be flexible. We get sick or life pulls us away. Rather than abandon our practice because we don't have an hour of time, we can dedicate five minutes and do what we can. If postures are inaccessible, we can breathe. If time is short, we can use our time wisely and still attend to the practice.

Even after decades of practicing yoga, there are days I do not want to show up. I force myself to my mat or my cushion. I observe my own resistance and accept that yoga is not always an easy choice. In the beginning, some changes may happen quickly. You notice muscles that are stronger, clothes fitting differently, or your mind becoming more tranquil. But after a while, the practice feels boring or uneventful. Keep in mind that yoga creates big changes over a long period of time. Yoga is not a quick fix that will take away your problems. Do not be discouraged when you practice and still have outside stress. Over time, your practice will allow you to manage life's challenges and teach you that the inner journey is always accessible. This path—this practice—requires dedication and effort. The fact that the practice asks you to show up for yourself over and over, even when you feel unworthy, makes it that much more meaningful.

DAY 67

There is nothing wrong with doing yoga with the intention to lose weight, strengthen your core, tone muscles, or increase flexibility. All of these physical benefits will come with a regular practice! You do not need to do difficult poses in order to see physical changes from yoga. Physical limitations need not deter you from showing up to your practice. Yoga is for *everyone*.

First and foremost, yoga is an inward journey. You are worthy of a personal practice that digs into your soul and asks how you would like to transform inside as well as out. Maybe you know what you want to change about yourself. Maybe you want clarity around a situation or relationship. Maybe you want support with an addiction or mental health issue. Maybe you are simply curious. All you need is a willingness to open your heart and your time to a practice that is for *you*. Then you can see what comes up.

Your practice can transform your body, mind, and soul. Your practice is an opportunity to show up for yourself and whatever healing it is you seek. There is a popular myth in our society that showing up for ourselves is selfish. If yoga is considered self-care, we feel guilty making space, and we quickly let our practice go when something *more important* arrives. In the midst of people needing you, responsibilities, and tasks, please take the time to show up for yourself. You are worth saving. You are worth a daily practice that will sustain and heal you. If you want to function best for everyone else, I firmly believe you have to put yourself first.

DAY 68

In Sanskrit, *sadhana* means "realization" and refers to our daily spiritual practice. Sadhana is both physical and spiritual. This has nothing to do with religion, although any religion you practice fits well into a yoga routine. Yoga doesn't ask you to believe in anything; yoga teaches that the answers are within you. Sadhana is our daily discipline, whether that's cleansing, meditating, prayer, physical practice, journaling, or being still. Sadhana is the practice that will lead us to realizations about who we are and what we're capable of. Regular sadhana takes care of our body and our mental state. Your own sadhana is reliable and safe, so when the outside world gets stressful or something huge occurs, you have your sadhana, your sacred practice, to ground and sustain you. This is why we create a regular sadhana. It is not only for when things are bad but also for when life is good. Sadhana grants access to our inner world, so we can make sense of the outside one. Your sadhana can look like waking, meditating, having tea, or journaling. Your sadhana can look like meditating and doing yoga at three in the afternoon. Sadhana is your practice and your realization.

DAY 69

Somewhere around the age of thirty-seven, I asked myself what I had done wrong. If life was supposed to look like marriage, a house, friends, family, evenly mowed grass, two cars, two kids, two careers—and I had all that—why did I feel so unsettled? And why did I need at least an entire bottle of wine to get through the night?

I had gathered all the things that were supposed to make me happy. I had mastered all the duties, kept all the balls in the air, and created an acceptable exterior. As problems arose, I found ways to quickly cope, such as shopping, substance abuse, poor eating, and charging ahead. I became very accustomed to running and numbing. I became very accustomed to propping everything up and ignoring myself. In building my world from the outside, I had no ability to move from my own heart. I reacted to life in order to survive, but I craved something that would fulfill and sustain me.

I finally returned to yoga, exhausted and desperate. I call it "spiritual surgery"—the moment of acknowledgment and the slow undoing in order to rediscover who we are at our center. You don't have to hit bottom in order to start. Maybe there has been illness, loss, or death. Maybe there is a persistent nagging, and you feel called to listen. Wherever you are, notice it. Then show up to your mat and tend to your practice. Your practice supports acknowledgment from the inside, which is always sustainable. Fulfillment does not happen as a result of a beautiful exterior; fulfillment happens when we turn inward, when we still the mind and gently ask, "*What longs to erupt from me?*"

DAY 70

As long as you keep moving forward, one step at a time, the destination will arrive. Actually, many destinations will arrive with many different paths to choose from along the way. It's like we are in a buffet line with unlimited tastes and sensations, and we can sample them all. There are not right or wrong choices. Anything you put on your plate has its own flavor, its own lesson. It is only through practice that we can eventually make the decisions to take what we like and reach for the things that align with our truth.

Along our path, during our many choices, endeavors, falls, and comebacks, we might feel alone as if we are failing and grasping or just doing our best to hang on. We observe other people who seem to float easily through life, and we wonder why it's so hard for us. Comparison turns our focus outward and provides a distorted view. Someone else's journey is none of our business. Direct your gaze inward to your body, your sensations, and your present experience. The most important journey—and the only one that needs tending to—is your inner journey. From a place of truth and integrity, we can make the best decisions for our outer circumstance. Only by truly knowing ourselves can we create and manifest our deepest desires. We learn through practice, not perfection. Make a choice and notice. Learn. Make a different choice and notice again. Let go of the expectation that you must move forward perfectly. Often, poor choices are the greatest teachers.

DAY 71

The miracle may not reveal itself when we are in the thick of it. We don't always see the light when we are in the middle of a dark time. We may struggle to find blessings in the midst of crisis. But for a moment, in a ray of sunshine, in a passing cloud, or in the perfectly gnarled branch of a tree, we sense that we are okay—that we are held. These moments of grace sustain us and inspire us to keep going, but we won't experience full realization until we fiercely and bravely walk the path as best we know how at that time.

Sometimes, our faith—faith in a higher power, faith in love, faith in ourselves—needs to be tested. Sometimes, this test arrives in the form of heartache and hardship. By walking the path anyway, by taking a step forward anyway, we are that much closer to being shown the miracle. Sometimes, walking forward looks like sitting still. When we've never been here before and we don't know the next right move, we can sit down. We can refrain from battling, pushing, and analyzing and just be. We can allow the grief of life to rise up inside of us, gnaw at our chest, and pour out of our bodies. We can be present for ourselves to feel, and that is the miracle. It is when we admit we do not know, when the blessing has yet to be revealed, and we stay.

DAY 72
Seated Cat/Cow

Arrive in your seat, either on the floor or in a chair. Place your hands on your knees, palms face down. Lengthen the spine, sitting up tall. Inhale and look up. Pull your heart forward and the shoulders back. Exhale as you lower your chin to your chest and curve the spine. Continue, front to back, arching and curving, inhaling as you arch, and exhaling as you curve. Allow the movement to grow. Your range of motion increases. Your breath lengthens and expands. You notice sensation building in temperature, in flexibility, and in letting go. The movement starts to feel intuitive and less like technique.

After several rounds of seated cat/cow, decide where to go next. You might want to draw circles with the torso one direction and then the other. You might want to stretch the arms up overhead or reach them onto the floor in front of you. Whatever your body craves, wherever your breath guides you, go there. Do that.

To begin our practice, we need to get a sense of what feels essential to the body in this moment. We are not always allowed to give ourselves exactly what we want in life. We can't always take a nap or go on vacation. In your space, during your practice, give yourself full permission. Honor the cravings with complete abandon. Let go of technique and rules. Begin lying down with hands on your belly. Begin standing up, and slowly move into downward-facing dog. This practice is yours, and it is an opportunity to give yourself exactly what you need. Yes, yoga is a discipline, but smiling and enjoying yourself are huge bonuses.

DAY 73

It's easy to walk the spiritual talk when life is good. Our hearts are whole. Our desires are being met. Our breath is easy. When life is hard, when the pain rises, your heart breaks, or your wishes seem to fade, is when the practice becomes the real teacher.

At Kripalu, the fifty-year-old mindfulness-based education center where I completed my teacher training, I learned about BRFWA, which stands for breathe, relax, feel, watch, and allow. BRFWA is a technique for riding difficult waves of sensation. Emotions move like waves. They arrive, build, crest, and fall. When I am in a difficult emotional state, it helps me to notice these waves and recognize that they always change, sometimes quickly, sometimes slowly. Using BFRWA allows us to have a full and real experience. Like the Sutras teach us, our ego wants to attach stories to every emotion; it's not the sensation that is so painful, but the story we attach. Our practice becomes learning to savor it all—the grief, the anger, and the frustration as well as the joy, the excitement, and the love.

There are many ways to jump off the wave before it gets too hard, such as denial, blaming, or numbing the sensation. But if we stay, if we ride the wave and ride through the pain, if we feel, watch, and allow, we will discover a myriad of things about ourselves. First, we will learn that we can survive difficult emotions. Second, we will discover that we will not, in fact break, or disappear as the result of pain. Lastly, we will realize there may be new insight we can take with us after seeing a difficult emotion through. When we stay, we arrive at the bottom of the wave as a new person.

DAY 74

The getting up was the hardest for me. Each time I tumbled from my sobriety, I felt the lowest I had ever felt. I felt hopeless, fearful, and full of doubt. Each time, begrudgingly, I reached out for a different kind of support. I added tools to the tool kit I already thought was too big.

The road of change is paved with many twists and turns. Our own perception of success and failure keeps us in turmoil when, actually, there may be nothing wrong. Really, if you are moving forward, if you are still showing up with curiosity, you are making progress. Making the choice to change something does not mean we will be perfect from then on out. We have willingness, but we still need practice. If we can allow setbacks to be teachers, we strengthen our resolve, and we increase our resilience. We improve our ability to succeed in the long run.

Setbacks are also great opportunities to treat ourselves with compassion. Our journey is cumulative, meaning any progress made is not lost if we temporarily revert to old behavior. The only true loss is if we give up completely, if we abandon our intention or our practice, and if we stop showing up to meet ourselves where we are. Remember that twists and turns are the price of growth. Being perfect from the start offers no wisdom, no chance to add new tools, and no chance to get back up. In the rising, we gain new perspectives. In the rising, we figure out the missing pieces. In the rising, and maybe most importantly, we learn that we *can*.

DAY 75

How is your practice going? Are you noticing progress? Is your confidence increasing? Are you getting bored? Throughout our practice, we will notice a range of sensations. Like the body, a playground of feelings and subtle longings, our practice will bring forth qualities. Some will be welcome and others deterring. We don't have to be quick to react to every nuance that arrives. When balance is off, there is no calamity. If you're tired, it doesn't mean there is anything to fix. A big part of your yoga practice is learning to be present with what is. Acceptance of the moment doesn't mean you have to like it. In fact, you don't need to label it at all. It's so hard to maintain a neutral perspective when we've been conditioned to assign labels to everything in our world. Somehow, assigning these labels gives us a sense of control. *If it's bad, change it. If it's good, hang on for dear life.*

We don't have as much control over the outside world as we think. Plus, something we label as bad could actually be good. We really don't know. Yoga teaches us that by observing and attending to our inner world, rather than judging the outside one, we achieve lessons in nonattachment, humility, compassion, and acceptance. We come to know that our inside practice affects our view of the outside, whether people or circumstances change or not. Our new perspective is not delusion. Actually, the illusion we have been living in, which says everything should look and feel a certain way, is removed. Thus, we can show up to our practice truly open, truly honest, and receive the benefits of quiet observation instead of harsh critique.

DAY 76

It's amazing how we can moan and groan about a choice we know must be made. Deep down, we always know. The best choice is not always the easy choice; many times, it is the hardest. Are you there? At the edge, wondering and shaking, and wondering if there is another way? Yes, there are challenges after you leap, but none are quite as exhilarating and terrifying as the initial jump.

I walked into my first recovery meeting. I told my boss I was quitting to be a stay-at-home mom. I called a therapist. I signed up for a writing class. I admitted to someone, "I love you." I made a point to say, "I'm sorry."

These are all things I've done that have made my stomach curl back in retaliation. My ego screams at me, *"No! This feels bad! This feels uncomfortable!"* I don't know about you, but I like feeling comfortable—warm, cozy, and secure. Maybe that's why difficult decisions, even in our best interest, are so hard to make. It's hard to stand up for ourselves. It's hard to ask for help. It's hard to put our heart out there in this loud, broken world.

Risk and fear look different for all of us. Maybe your greatest fear is someone else's comfort zone. Maybe some fears are universal and shared among all of us, such as loneliness, abandonment, and rejection. Maybe we all have a fear of ourselves and what we're actually capable of. If you are out of your comfort zone, place a hand on your heart and pay attention. There is goodness, greatness, and even amazement heading your way. Take the leap.

DAY 77

One way yogis believed we reach enlightenment is through death. When we die, we are reunited with Brahman, the creator and source of all things. One way to reach *samadhi* (liberation and enlightenment) while alive is by renouncing everything worldly—all possessions, all people, all ways of culture and society. Monks and nuns renunciate earthly desires and attachments in order to live closer to God. This is their practice. Gandhi, Buddha, and many yogis were also renunciates.

Most of us do not want to leave our families, conveniences, pleasures, jobs, or society in order to experience liberation. How nice that Patanjali, credited with writing the Yoga Sutras, offers a way to reach enlightenment while still remaining part of the modern world.

The third way to reach enlightenment is through our daily practice. Patanjali states that when we bring certain qualities to our practice, we move closer to *Atman*, our true, inner Self. We need faith, a belief in ourselves or in something outside ourselves. We need vigor, the energy to show up ready and willing. We need memory to learn our lessons. We need contemplation to be still, be curious, and ask questions. We need discernment to be nonjudgmental and to distinguish between the false ego and Atman.[16] With these qualities, or even a few of them, embedded in our daily practice, we feel freer, lighter, and more at peace. We don't need to live as a monk or renunciate. We can show up, practice nonjudgment, learn from our past, and remain open and curious. We can live enlightened every day.

....

16. Satchidananda, *The Yoga Sutras of Patanjali*, 35.

DAY 78

The Sutras talk a lot about faith as a necessary part of a yoga practice. This can be a real turnoff for many people who think *faith* refers to a religious belief. Yes, the word *faith* is used in our society when referring to someone's religion, but *faith* also means trust in something we do not know or cannot see. Faith becomes a practice in showing up, not something we worship. *Sraddha*, the Sanskrit word for "faith," also translates to "sincerity."[17] We practice yoga with the faith that we will learn something new about ourselves or the world. We are sincere in our practice, seeking truth and an end to our illusion. We have no agenda or ill will. We trust our bodies and the process. We keep showing up to our practice. Faith is necessary to keep going, and our effort is sincere.

When Patanjali talks about faith, he also means courage.[18] It takes courage to continually show up, especially for something we can't see. Luckily, the physical practice of yoga yields many tangible benefits, such as changes in our bodies. The intangible, subtle benefits, such as releasing energy and changing our character, require a more attuned perspective. Maybe you feel friendlier or kinder after you do yoga. Maybe you are more patient and accepting. Do not dismiss these qualities as coincidence or chance. Your loving-kindness toward yourself and your practice has no choice but to ripple out to other people and projects in your life. Yoga is physical and spiritual. Like the muscles that change, *you* also change.

....

17. Satchidananda, *The Yoga Sutras of Patanjali*, 35.
18. Satchidananda, *The Yoga Sutras of Patanjali*, 35.

DAY 79

Dedication to your practice begins like planting a seed. You prepare, make space, set your alarm, and show up regularly. At first, you don't notice much, but slowly you begin to see changes. You ache less. You have more energy. Postures change. You can balance longer or fold a little deeper. You begin to see lessons from yoga in your life. The practice starts to seep into work, relationships, and casual encounters. You are more flexible when things don't go your way. You accept detours and setbacks. You remember to breathe before you act. You consider yourself before answering a question.

When a seed starts growing, it is underground and unseen, and your practice is the same. Although there is no flower yet, much is changing. Important roots are forming, ensuring a strong base. The process takes time. A flower does not bloom mere days after the seed is planted. We accept this process of nature. Yet we expect something very different from ourselves and our practice. We want immediate results. We cannot afford to waste time; we want change now. Swami Kripalu stated, "Patience is a key virtue on the path of yoga. It often eludes us because of its simplicity, yet it forms the foundation of a true yogi's practice."[19] I agree. Patience might be simple, but it's not easy, especially in today's world of instant gratification. Anything meaningful and sustainable takes time. Allow your practice to grow from simple seed to breathtaking flower. Stay patient. Stay with your practice. When the flower blooms, it will be that much more special.

....
19. Levitt, *Pilgrim of Love*, 182.

DAY 80
Cat / Cow

Begin on your hands and knees. Tighten your core slightly in order to stabilize the pelvis and lengthen the spine. Notice the tailbone reaching back and the crown of your head pointing ahead. As you inhale, let your belly drop and the tailbone tilt upward. Observe how the pelvis responds when the belly drops. As you exhale, pull the belly up and back. The tailbone will tuck, and the spine will curve. Continue to move through cat/cow at a slow pace. Let the breath guide the movement, signaling when to let the belly drop and fill with breath and when to squeeze the belly back as you empty. Allow your eyes to close. Notice when you close your eyes, the outside world disappears, and you are automatically brought within. The body feels different. The mind feels different. Sensations feel more noticeable. Hands on the mat. Knees on the mat. Breath in the belly.

Cat/cow can be done every day for years and always feel a little different. The movement is an excellent way to warm up the spine, but it also helps create introversion and insight. Cat/cow is a great posture to make meditative. With eyes closed and a focus on the breath, the movement starts to feel intuitive, like our body is making the choice and not our mind. We become the observer of this, and we watch the mind watching the body. We watch the breath happening and the body responding. Our body might feel like expanding the movement by folding into child's pose or lifting into upward dog. When our practice cultivates this introspection and we spend intimate time with the Knower, we achieve a real calmness in our Self.

DAY 81

Yoga is a lifelong practice that is accessible to any *body*. The image of yoga according to most media gives the impression that a yoga practice is for a certain body—a young body, a flexible body, or an athletic body. The truth is: yoga provides benefits even when physical limitations prevent you from doing certain postures. A more challenging posture does not necessarily provide greater benefit than an easier one. You can build strength in your core while standing in mountain pose just as well as holding plank. Balance comes whether your hand is on the back of a chair for support or not. Flexibility comes from consistency and showing up, however your body is best able. For many, the more gentle, slower postures can be more challenging than a "big" pose or a fast-moving flow. A lot of us have more trouble being still or moving slowly than pushing and rushing ourselves through.

If you are able, it's important to move the spine all six directions before starting your practice (front to back, side to side, right twist, and left twist). This increases synovial fluid, which cushions the joints and vertebra. Or maybe moving the spine *is* your practice. Yoga does not require that you hop from seated to standing throughout the practice. Progress is noticeable after consistent practice. You may notice greater range of motion in your shoulders or deeper twists or folds. You may notice the ability to take deeper breaths. Your body is a magnificent system of bones, joints, muscles, and tendons. An accessible practice will support your body, wherever it's at, for the rest of your life.

DAY 82

As a recovering people pleaser, I am careful to respect my own needs and desires while still being helpful and kind. Constantly saying "yes" and living for the sake of others seems nice, but it will lead to resentment, frustration, and a lack of self-awareness. When we don't honor ourselves, we become agitated, depressed, and indifferent. It's okay to be easygoing, but we don't want to swing too far and become victim to everyone else and every life circumstance that comes our way.

Our desires change over time, so if you feel chaotic or unmotivated throughout your day, reassess your values. Make a list and determine if your time is well spent according to who you are today. In no particular order, my values are: family, writing, teaching, and my inner growth. When I first saw my values laid out on paper, I realized how much time I spent in areas that didn't support my truth. I noticed my old definition of success kept me overworked in the wrong profession. I saw how accepting social obligations I no longer cared about prevented me from doing yoga or spending time with my kids. By letting go of what didn't support my current values, I was able to shift my life into one that served me and therefore everyone else.

I still get caught up in the people-pleasing. I worry what people think and expect of me, and I have trouble saying "no." Putting myself and my values first allows me to make healthier decisions and leads to less frustration. If something no longer aligns with your values, it's time to lovingly let it go.

DAY 83

Sometimes, when I stare ahead, I literally get ahead of myself. I want everything to change at once, and am overwhelmed by the long road in front of me. The year I knew everything needed to change, I had no idea where to begin. My life was so out of hand. I was raising babies, teaching full time, and commuting far into the city. I was running my own business. I was drinking too much in order to cope. My husband and I were fighting and struggling. It was too much to admit all the pieces were falling apart, so I started small. I signed up for yoga. My small town had just opened a studio, and I bought a monthly pass. I showed up on my mat, and I breathed. That was my only undertaking—to breathe for the entire hour and a half.

When you feel like everything is too much, choose one small thing, and let that be enough. Doing one small thing *can* change your life. The greatest part is—you don't have to know where the new thing will lead you. Looking back, that mat and that studio became my sacred space to connect with myself and my intuition. So, a few years later, when I really needed to face hard decisions, I had my practice to guide and support me. What is one small thing you can do for now? Watch in wonderment as your one small thing creates larger ripples and, eventually, entire shifts in your life you hadn't even considered.

DAY 84

Dharana means "focus," and it is the sixth of the Eight Limbs of Yoga. The Eight Limbs of Yoga include eight practices to support a fulfilled and purposeful life. Dharana comes right after presence and right before meditation. In our busy lives, it's natural to lose focus. We have an easily lured, happily distracted mind. Our mind loves wandering through the aisles of Target, the pet store, the gas station, or wherever we find ourselves wandering. The last thing the mind wants to do is sit still. If we spend too much time unfocused, we are more easily distracted, we make mistakes, and we feel unsettled even after completing tasks.

On the days we are the busiest, achieving focus during our practice is that much harder to do. My mind taunts me, *"You can't do yoga today. I can give you ten things to get up and do **right now** that are more important than sitting here trying to meditate."*

As convincing as the mind can be, remember that stillness and your practice are exactly what you need when you feel pulled in many directions. Get still and bring your attention to the breath. Sometimes, closing the eyes with an active mind can be too much, and it helps to focus on an object in front of us, such as a candle or a picture. Hold your attention on your breath or the object. It might take one deep inhale. It might take ten deep inhales. Notice if the voice in your head becomes quieter. After a few minutes holding focus, you will be more prepared to tackle the day and less likely to lose your attention throughout.

DAY 85

Truth is revealed in seemingly empty spaces—the unspoken words, the breath, the silence. When we create space, we see our own truth more clearly, and we are able to hear the truth of others. When was the last time you felt the permission of space? Our society is like one giant hoarder, and there is no space left to listen or to be. In the constant noise, there is no reality, only illusion and distraction. We drag around the residue of old wounds and relationships. We bend our heads over phones and computers. We expose our minds to continuous information, and we carelessly grab for pieces that will save us.

Our minds are so full and so loud that our own inner wisdom gets completely buried. To access this wisdom—to access ourselves—we need to pay attention to the spaces that exist in our practice. There is a slight rising before folding the body over. There is one more breath to sustain us before we come out of a pose. My chest shakes after each heart opener, fearful of what has been jostled loose from the depths and brought to the surface. I have a sense it's every lost relationship, every heartache, and every buried resentment.

Create space for yourself. And create space for someone else. Holding space for another person is powerful—sometimes more powerful than inserting our voice or advice. In relationships, we can listen to someone else and offer silence instead of trying to fix the problem. Spaces exist in life, and we don't have to fill them. There is truth, love, and tenderness in the seemingly empty spaces.

DAY 86

A yoga practice can certainly be led by a teacher, done in a certain order, and focused on proper alignment. But a one-size yoga practice does not fit all. Different bodies and personalities, as well as different life experiences, might benefit from different practices. There was a time in my twenties, when I was new to the techniques and postures, that I took Ashtanga yoga and completed the ninety-minute series, which included the same postures, in the same order, every single time. I memorized the Sanskrit names and directions. My body imprinted the feeling of arriving in each pose. The discipline of Ashtanga yoga teaches stamina, cultivates presence, and allows the thoughts in the mind to shift into the background as you move through the series.

Sometimes, we need discipline. I loved showing up to my Ashtanga class and felt accomplished when I left. But there are also times when we can benefit from more choice and agency in our practice, and yoga allows for this as well. A personal yoga practice focused on choices, rather than discipline, that also gives permission and responds compassionately to the body can be empowering if your choices have been taken away. Practicing self-awareness and responsibility during a personal yoga practice removes victimhood and gives you back control. Honoring your body on the mat adds to self-love and self-forgiveness. You are no longer at someone else's mercy. Your practice on the mat strengthens your ability to choose for yourself in life. Your practice is a reflection and a teacher for whatever you need. Embrace each choice as a message from your soul, and trust that your choice is always right.

DAY 87

Play is an important part of our practice. We can get bogged down by any spiritual discipline and start to take ourselves too seriously. Humans are gifted the innate ability to find joy in the midst of hardship and beauty in the mundane. Think of a time you have been crying and simultaneously laughing. We hold the capacity to screw up and then laugh at ourselves. We recognize the absurdity when life gets turned upside down, yet we know at our center that we contain joy.

Play reminds us it's okay to let go, to loosen our grip on perfectly maintained routines and practices, to let go of our need to stay in control, and to become unattached to the things we *think* are keeping us stable. Play is part of our true nature. It is smiling when we fall out of balance and laughing when the tears threaten to arrive. To experience joy in the moment *is* a spiritual practice. It's called presence, and even if the larger world is coming apart, this moment can be a good one. Play in the midst of pain is one of the greatest healers. When we access our joy, we access our unshakable Self. We are reminded that we are still in there, and nothing can touch our infinite joy and playfulness, even if we're a bit lost right now. The discipline does not define our path. Instead, it supports it—even when we're out just having fun.

DAY 88

How would you behave differently if you knew it would all work out? Would you write the book? Would you apply for the job? Would you take the trip? What would it look like to go all in? In the relationship, in the adventure, in the career?

A good amount of pause, caution, and humility is healthy. But I have a feeling we sabotage ourselves more than we need to. I have a feeling we let fear talk us out of something we really want. I have a feeling we become paralyzed because of our own self-doubt.

Regularly, I hear people say things like, "I always wanted to _____."

And I think, *"Why haven't you?"*

Sometimes, I imagine a world where everyone goes after their dreams unapologetically and with great fervor. We have this one life. We have gifts and talents that are uniquely ours. We are here for a purpose, and that purpose is to not look like everyone else. Your dreams are not an accident, and they matter—*you* matter.

What if it all goes right? How would you move forward if you knew your doubts and excuses were imaginary? At least most of them are. Sure, there will be roadblocks along the way, but the obstacles are only signs pointing you another way, a way you hadn't considered and a way that may even be better than your original plan. You won't know unless you go after it and with the faith that it all works out.

DAY 89

I learn the most about myself when I've had a long week when everything goes wrong or the unexpected happens. When I had a plan, and I had to throw my plan out. As parents, caregivers, siblings, and friends, the unexpected happens. Someone gets sick. Loved ones need our help, so we adjust. Normally, being there for others is manageable and part of life, but sometimes, everything happens at once. Your sister and mom both need something on the same day. You have a deadline at work and are already busier than usual. You haven't gotten enough sleep. Appointments and commitments have piled up, and you are suddenly very stressed out.

Your yoga practice seems the easiest to discard, even when it might be what you need most. Sometimes, all we need is to acknowledge ourselves. I know when I am overextended because I get very crabby, and I start to blame everything out in the world. My kindness disappears, and I have problems with the economy, politics, drivers, and strangers at the store.

Take a deep breath, and let it out with an audible sigh or even a scream. Inhale again. On the exhale, sigh loudly or make a sound. Do it again. And again. Let the exhale cleanse you, and let whatever sound emerges free you. When the week or month has been long and you feel yourself bubbling over, drag yourself to your mat and breathe. Let yourself sigh, and let yourself shake. The days our practice would truly serve us are often the days we try to avoid. We get used to feeling bad and are unmotivated to find solutions. Inhale and sigh it out. Your practice is powerful and worth it.

DAY 90
Legs Up the Wall

Lay your mat perpendicular to a wall. Begin sitting sideways with a shoulder touching the wall. Lean back and swing your legs up the length of the wall. Try to get your seat as close to the wall as possible, ideally touching. It can take a bit to maneuver the body into this posture, but it is worth it! Once your legs are up the wall, lay the upper body down. Place your hands on your belly, bend the arms overhead, or rest your arms at your sides. Allow the muscles in the legs to loosen and relax. Don't lock out the knees, and keep the ankles soft. If your legs start to tingle or shake, try putting a blanket or bolster between your seat and the wall. Stay here for five, ten, or fifteen minutes. To come out of the pose, place your feet on the wall and roll onto a side in a fetal position. Breathe here. Let the spine and body reset.

Legs up the wall is my favorite yoga pose. It is refreshing anytime I feel tired, calming when I feel stressed, and relaxing after a long day. When my physical body aches, especially the low back, legs up the wall is my go-to. If you've been sitting or driving for a long stretch, try this restorative pose. Legs up the wall improves circulation, calms the nervous system, relieves low back pain, and restores balance to body and mind. For swollen ankles, varicose veins, and skin issues, legs up the wall can help. Remember that your practice does not have to be active. Knowing what your body needs and offering it a restorative posture is still yoga.

DAY 91

By observing the activities of the ego, we learn a lot about ourselves. We see how the ego works, and we become aware of the other part of us: the true, real Self. The simplest way to discern ego from Self is to look at our motivation. Ego is always motivated by fear—the fear, as Eckhart Tolle writes, "of being nobody, the fear of nonexistence, the fear of death."[20]

A lot of times we think of the ego in terms of pride, cockiness, or self-righteousness, but these bolstering qualities also stem from fear, fear of not being enough or never having enough.

The ego will convince you that buying a new car will make you feel better or that an intimate partner will save you. The ego is constantly in a battle with fear, telling us false ways to complete ourselves. When we listen to the ego, we only make things worse. A new car does not fulfill us, so we need more and more.

Developing an intimate relationship with our ego increases our awareness of Self. The ego does not need to be eliminated or ignored. It simply needs to be watched and discerned. If we check our motivations behind our actions, we will be less disappointed when they don't fulfill the ego's false promises. Likewise, when we become aware of the ego and can call it out, the ego has less power over us. We think and act according to truth instead of illusion. We make more informed decisions. Watch your ego; get intimate with the ways it wants you to stay in fear.

....
20. Tolle, *A New Earth*, 80.

DAY 92

Like many journeys, a yoga practice begins with an intention, something hopeful or maybe something painful within the Self. In the end, the more you practice, the more you learn yoga is not only about how we treat ourselves but also how we treat all of our relationships, society, and the world. Yoga makes you a better person—not because you're perfect but because you've awakened compassion within you.

Yoga teaches us to acknowledge our progress. Consider your journey so far and how your practice has allowed you to be more compassionate and proud of the road you've traveled. Acknowledge your progress. I hope you have noticed changes in yourself. Maybe others have noticed these changes as well. Yoga not only heals the person practicing. Yoga heals every person, relationship, and circumstance the practicing yogi touches. For every happy ending, there is a brave journey that came before, and when we show up for ourselves, amazing shifts happen as a result of our self-acknowledgment. We are brave enough to try. We are brave enough to change. We are faithful enough to keep going. The more you dig into who you are, during a posture or a silent morning, the more you give others permission to grow and change through their journeys. The practice you have created for yourself is an accomplishment worth recognizing. Your practice has set your intention in motion and probably brought other gifts. Life and all its surprises may seem more manageable now because you have your practice as a foundation. Well done.

PRACTICE 4
Breath (Pranayama)

B reath is powerful. In yoga philosophy, breath is more than a physical function of the body. Breath is the energy that connects us to the Divine—the truth. Pranayamas were the original yoga practice from five thousand years ago and are still part of yoga today. Consider this: our breath is the only autonomic function of the body we can control. We cannot control the heartbeat, function of organs, or digestion, but we can restrain and elongate the breath. If we don't think about breathing, it happens on its own as a normal part of our body. By practicing different pranayamas (breath techniques), we change the nervous system and our state of mind. We also connect with our true Self. We reach liberation, awakening, purpose, and joy. Prana is an aliveness that pulses within, breathing heart and soul into our daily efforts and pursuits. Prana awakens our senses and feeds our inner desire. Prana invites us to ask our heart, rather than our head. Let's dive in!

DAY 93

The path of yoga is a path to enlightenment. If there is an end goal to why people practice yoga, enlightenment is it. I don't know if I know what enlightenment is, although I agree with many of my teachers that my practice has led me to moments of freedom and pure awareness. Historically, people began practicing yoga as a way to overcome suffering. The human experience is full of suffering from inside our own mind to external injustices and tragedies. As a result of suffering, yogis sought practices to make sense of the human experience. They sought a path to truth and the Divine not only in death but in life. Pranayama is a way to understand our holiness and our connectedness, so our experience on this path is not so lonely, confusing, or unhappy.

Yogis practiced pranayamas because the breath techniques gave them illuminating experiences about what it means to be human. If we break down the word *pranayama* in Sanskrit, *prana* means "breath," *yama* means "restraint," and *ayama* means "length." Thus, *pranayama* means "to restrain or lengthen the breath." Pranayama is not only breathing. Pranayamas are breath techniques that "increase pranic capacity" and are practiced with the intention to change our awareness.[21] Yogis have experienced healing, wholeness, and transformation of the body and mind through continued practice of pranayama. At the least, the breath calms you down, but breath can also lead you to an enlightening experience of your own.

....
21. Muktibodhananda, *Hatha Yoga Pradipika*, 682, 710.

DAY 94

Another name for pranayama is "aliveness." So, when we cultivate prana, we increase our aliveness. What does it feel like to be alive? We are more joyful, even in the midst of pain. We are grateful and can see our abundance. We don't hide negative feelings, but we know of our true nature, our state of love.

Imagine prana as water in a glass. We want the glass to be full, but as we go about our day and our life, our energy—our *aliveness*—gets depleted. People hurt us. We endure tragedy or loss. Someone cuts us off while driving. We don't get the job we want. We have a fight with our partner. The glass becomes emptier and emptier. One way pranayamas work is to increase our aliveness, to fill our cup. We increase prana by noticing the breath. Each time you practice yoga and meditation, each time you observe the breath or match your breath with a movement, you increase prana. When prana is full, we feel alive.

We all know what it feels like to be tired and empty. We struggle just to go through the motions, acting on autopilot and without awareness. We react to life rather than direct our energy from a place of intention and truth. We are indifferent and uncaring. Conversely, having our prana cup full deepens our connection to our intuition, so we behave from a state of love and tolerance rather than ego. Connected to our truth, we are less likely to react out of fear or frustration. With prana, life becomes more manageable because we have shifted our energy from depletion and reaction to aliveness and awareness.

DAY 95

In addition to providing us with energy and aliveness, prana also connects us to our true Self. Humans are excellent at avoiding pain, shifting responsibility, stuffing emotions, and denying. Pranayamas loosen the sludge that hasn't been dealt with. Pranayamas are like rakes that dredge our insides in order to be clean. When we practice breathing, we allow buried hurts or misperceptions to rise up in order to be addressed and released.

Your mind does not need to be involved. Practicing a pranayama can unearth and let go of something toxic in your body, and you don't ever have to know it happened. This is because prana has to do with the nonrational part of us; prana is our link to the Divine, the Divine outside of us and the Divine that *is* us. You can call this divine part of yourself intuition, inner knowing, pure love, or essence. The part of us that is not the mind, not our thoughts, is prana. Prana is the energy that moves all things. Experiences, possessions, beliefs, and appearance have nothing to do with prana. When there is stress, outside turmoil, or inner hurt, prana is the healing life force that brings you back to your true state. Yogis know this because with consistent breath practice, they have reached states of pure awareness, peace, and joy. Pranayamas remove the veil, so you can experience the joy of being exactly who you are. You might call this awareness enlightenment. Regardless of the name, prana makes inner peace and contentment possible.

DAY 96

Are you angry, muddy, or confused? Try some *kapalabhati* (skull-shining breath). Kapalabhati cleanses the nasal passages and the soul. It tones and strengthens abdominal muscles and helps reduce constipation. Like all pranayamas, kapalabhati activates intuition, so you might feel clearer afterward and more focused. Subtle sensations that may happen as a result of this breath practice are feelings of physical lightness, less brain fog, and less heaviness in the belly and gut. Like polishing unused silver to reveal its shiny surface, this powerful breath practice rids the body of dust and grime, and it brings an ethereal lightness to the mind.

You might want to grab a tissue or clear your nose before this practice. To begin, exhale forcefully out the nose and pull the belly back toward the spine. As soon as the inhale arrives, exhale again out the nose. On the inhale, the belly expands but without your effort. The exhale is your effort; the inhale is the result. Do this several times, focusing only on the exhale. Start with ten rounds, and increase to fifteen, twenty, or more. You can place a hand on your belly to feel it pulling back on the exhale and softly expanding on the inhale.

After several rounds, return to normal breathing. Watch the breath as it comes back. Notice if anything has shifted, and observe sensations. The breath evens out. The heartbeat slows down. Pay attention to the body, remembering it is your teacher. States of mind and awareness are brought to the center, and we sense a different Self. With kapalabhati, something has just been removed, and something new is here.

DAY 97

It's common to get used to a certain routine or way of doing things, and one of the best lessons from yoga is that we can always grow, change, and adjust. The practice changes, and we change. Life changes, and we need to shift our expectations. We get an injury or become ill, and our practice doesn't look like we intended. When the body has a setback, it's easy to get disappointed or down on ourselves. But no matter what it looks like, we can still do yoga.

At the heart of yoga is the breath. Breath takes us into our bodies and into our hearts. The poses have many physical benefits, and when we add breath, the benefits increase. Regardless of the difficulty of a pose, the single-pointed focus on breath during a yoga practice allows our mind to shift from thoughts to sensations. The mind lets go of past or future worry and moves to present attention. So, you see, while we are practicing specific pranayamas, which all have specific benefits and purposes, you do not need to complicate your practice. Be careful if your mind is shifting to thoughts like "*I can't do this. I don't understand this. I'm doing it wrong.*" Go easy on yourself, and don't let your critical mind creep back in just because you're learning something new. Simply watching the breath, as we have been doing from the start, will bring clarity and improved health for body and mind. While there are many pranayama techniques, any attention on the breath during your practice provides benefits. Continue observing the breath as you practice poses and while you meditate. This new, simple attention on breath goes a long way.

DAY 98

The original yogis used breath as a way to move deeper into the layers of Self, to travel beneath the surface of outside noise and distraction, to uncover buried emotions and sensations, and to sit in the place of truth. Yogis believe the breath is the thread that connects the body, mind, and soul and that it is the portal to our true essence. A human being's essence is our divinity and our purpose. When we travel to the depths of our being, we sit a little easier, we sleep without disturbance, and we breathe and remain present throughout our day. We might discover something painful or revelatory, but the main benefit from breath practices is that they simply bring us ease.

Of course if we go even further, breath practices can increase our productivity, clarity, and performance. Proper breath helps us work better, participate in sports better, handle relationships better, and live from a place of authenticity and joy. I've said that breath is connected to joy, and what I mean is joy of spirit, not necessarily happiness or a life of no problems. Breath will not eliminate life's struggles, but it will shift your inner state to a place of more acceptance.

Imagine planting a garden and breathing deeply, intentionally. Imagine swinging a golf club with a full, balanced breath. Imagine holding a difficult conversation with someone and breathing first to gain the best words. Breath can help us in our day-to-day as much as it helps us on our inward journey. By practicing mindful breathing during yoga, we not only feel better during our yoga practice—we also move differently in life.

DAY 99

In a yoga class, it's common to hear people breathing. During your practice, you are able to sense your own breath in feeling and in sound. *Ugayi* is a pranayama that means "ocean-sounding breath." Some people refer to this breath as Darth Vader because of the audible exhale. Like waves on the ocean, ugayi is calming, even, and cleansing.

To practice, bring the palm of your hand to face your mouth, like it is a mirror. Inhale through the nose. Then exhale out of an open mouth, and fog up the mirror. Feel the exhale on your palm. Do this a few times, and notice the restriction at the back of your throat in order to fog up the mirror. Also notice the sound, that ocean sound. Notice the length, slow and even. Now, close your mouth on the exhale, but keep the sensation of fogging up a mirror in the back of the throat. Keep the ocean sound. Ugayi is done completely through the nose but with restriction at the back of the throat on the exhale.

The sound enough is calming. Ugayi focuses on the exhale, ensuring a complete emptying. Ugayi is practiced during yoga classes because it draws the yogi inward and keeps a single-pointed focus on your breath, both with sound and physical sensation. Let the breath carry you as you exhale and fold. Your concentration will increase, and your nervous system will respond. You will feel calmer and move deeper into your practice. Emotions beneath the surface will be more apparent, and after several minutes, or an hour, you will feel like you have traveled to a different place, a place inside yourself, where there is much wisdom.

DAY 100

When I was at my yoga teacher training, there was a specific tree I always went to on my breaks. I took a blanket and spread it across the grass by the exposed roots at its base. I sat down, propped myself right up against the tree's trunk, and leaned my head back against the rough, jagged bark. I took full, deep breaths. I breathed in the prana and the wisdom of this solid, undeterred force of nature.

I believe in the wisdom of nature because I feel calm and peaceful when I'm in it. My body seems to have a response of "*I am home.*" I believe in all the lessons we can glean from trees that endure weather and society and time. I believe if we lean on nature, like I leaned on that tree, we not only remember who we are, but we receive the answers we need. We remember that we *are* the tree—the roots, the earth, the branches, and the wind between the leaves. We remember that like the tree, we can stand tall—no matter what threatens to shake us or make us snap. All we have to do is ask. The tree spoke to me, and I heard what it said.

To spend time in nature is to acknowledge our connection. The prana that exists within us is the same life force that exists in all living things. Instead of overlooking the natural world or taking it for granted, we can walk on the grass, admire passing clouds, and lean on a tree. We can breathe in fresh air and notice flitting birds.

Ask for guidance. You'll be surprised when nature speaks. Listen.

DAY 101

Breath is the physical inhale and exhale. It is also an energy we can't quite describe. Taking deep breaths expands lung capacity, which is why we are able to do physical activities more successfully with proper breath. Breathing also improves our mental state. It is common advice to "take a few deep breaths" when we feel stressed or out of alignment with life. Deep breaths have a direct effect on the nervous system, and we feel calmer and more at ease.

Activating prana also increases the energy of spirit within us. So, in addition to breathing more fully and helping our physical body, we awaken the layers of spiritual energy that make us feel more alive and remind us we are more than a physical body; we are also energy. The simplicity of watching or holding the breath enlivens this energy, so we are more able to access the truth of our divinity. Practicing pranayamas deepens our connection to the part of ourselves that is connected to the Universe and all living things. When we understand this connection, we come closer to a sensation of enlightenment and internal peace.

Additionally, deep breathing clears negativity and rids us of the illusion that we are separate. Through breath, we sense we are part of a bigger whole. Yogis called this bigger part of us Brahman and believed pranayamas helped us understand that we are the drop and also the entire ocean. The drop cannot be separate from the ocean. Yoga practices, including breathing, were thought to bring humans closer to Brahman, the divine part of every living being. Inhale and breathe in the energy of all things; exhale and become the entire ocean.

DAY 102

The Sutras don't actually talk much about specific breathing techniques or pranayamas. Patanjali mentions the breath as a powerful and necessary part of yoga but only as a straightforward practice in being mindful of the inhale and the exhale. What he does say about the breath is that it is directly linked to the mind. Hatha yoga and Buddhist traditions hold the same view. As we know, prana is breath and life force. Watching the breath increases prana, the energy that flows upward and outward in the body and connects us to our intuition and lighter states. The opposite of prana is *apana*, the energy that flows downward in the body and regulates menstruation, digestion, and elimination. According to the Sutras, "The aim is to bring together the prana and apana."[22] We want these energies balanced.

When we breathe evenly, with an equal length inhale and an equal length exhale, prana increases and moves up while apana moves down. These two energies are like a seesaw, and both affect each other. When prana and apana are balanced, we feel balanced. Balance is achieved just by watching the inhale and exhale, allowing prana and apana to meet in the middle. There is no magical or complicated technique. Breathing evenly simply activates prana and apana, and the body and mind are brought to union. *Yoga* means "union" or "to yoke," so it's interesting that this simple concept of prana and apana, of uniting and balancing these two energies in the body, explains the purpose of our entire yoga practice.

....
22. Satchidananda, *The Yoga Sutras of Patanjali*, 54.

DAY 103

Our outer journeys—the relationships we cultivate, the families we care for, the careers we sustain, and our day-to-day efforts—are meaningful. Our inner journey, however, is often forgotten, as we are constantly pulled by the necessities of everyday life. We may dedicate a short time to our practice, but 99 percent of the time, we are in motion, taking care of things, thinking about things, and living our lives. We need our logical, thinking mind; it keeps us organized, oriented, and dedicated to our day.

The greatest part of yoga is that we can practice all the time—during our normal day and in all our relationships. Yes, we need our logical mind throughout our day, but we also need prana, which means moving according to our heart and intuition. Prana moves us to a place of deep sensation, whether emotional or physical. An example of moving from prana might be calling someone to say, "I love you." It might be hugging your child or a family member. Prana lets you know when something is off. It's like that icky feeling in your gut. When moved by prana, we speak up. We let go of work, and we play or go for a walk. We finally make time for ourselves. We get to the art project or cook a delicious meal. We are less pulled by outcome and more motivated by heart.

Of course we need to rely on rational thought to complete tasks and interact with the human world. But we also need prana—moments of divine interception when we are moved into sensation and allowed to feel. We are in our mind enough. That sweetness, and all that is dear to you, is prana, and prana keeps you alive.

DAY 104

Even though emotions are physical as sensation, we really don't know what to do with an emotion until we rationalize it through our mind. If we are sad, we cry or lash out. If we are angry, we might isolate or cancel plans. If we are happy, we smile and call a friend.

At some point during adolescence, we learned to name and label our emotions. We became accustomed to defining an emotion based on an occurrence with no regard for what the body may be feeling.

Often during a counseling session, when talking about something that disturbs me, my therapist will ask, "Where do you feel that in your body?" It took me some time to consider that the emotion *was* actually somewhere in my body and could be felt at all. *What does sadness feel like as sensation? How is it different from frustration? Am I sad?* What if you didn't name the emotion first but felt it instead? Sadness might feel different in the body depending on what caused it. The sensation of sadness might not feel the same every single time, and it might not require the same reaction. In fact, emotions might not need any reaction at all. Yoga teaches us that emotions simply need to be felt. Once felt, they will move, and new sensations will arrive to pique our curiosity.

Stay in the body. Yes, our mind will help us take action if necessary, but it's possible for the body to move through an emotion without ever naming it. Breathing helps us stay with emotions without the need to label them or react. We tackle the emotion in our body and may never need to disturb the mind.

DAY 105

Despite any of our experiences, we are a body connected to an energetic being and, yes, connected to a state of joy. When our body is connected with heart, soul, and truth, we can experience joy even if something bad or tragic is happening in our outside world. Breath connects us to our true state. It gets us out of our head, which doesn't always give us an accurate portrayal of our experience.

Just like the tree is not dependent on anything outside of itself to remain a tree, our Self is not dependent on external people, places, or circumstances.

Consider a time when you exercised, did yoga, or meditated or a time you went to a concert, ran through a rainstorm, or laughed really hard with friends. After any of these experiences, you may have felt freer, lighter, and more joyful. Even if something uncomfortable was playing out in your life, you were able to glimpse your true state of joy despite external chaos. This is the energy of prana.

Practices that use breath in order to bring us deeper into our body remind us of this true state of being and are helpful when the world has us too much in our head. *Place your hand on your heart, and notice the rise and fall of your chest as you breathe. What sensations do you notice?* Maybe you notice the air entering and leaving the nostrils or the lifting and lowering of the heart space beneath your hand.

There is a rhythm inside, and it's more than the beat of your heart. The rhythm is energy and a connection to your truest state.

DAY 106

Some of the most helpful findings on how breath can help with stress come from research on trauma, namely, how the nervous system responds after a traumatic event and how breath affects the system. Bessel van der Kolk, author of *The Body Keeps the Score*, cites heart rate variability as a key indictor of how someone is able to deal with stress. Heart rate variability measures how the nervous system responds to breathing. Based on his findings, van der Kolk states that "lack of fluctuation in heart rate in response to breathing, not only has negative effects on thinking and feeling, but also how the body responds to stress."[23] Similar research on how coherent breathing has helped victims of trauma, conducted by Richard P. Brown and Patricia L. Gerbarg, also shows how the breath increases our stress resilience, and Brown and Gerbarg write that breathing increases "the capacity to recover and rebound from challenging events."[24] With breath, we can teach the nervous system to be more flexible and resilient.

It seems almost too simple that breath can balance the body and eliminate symptoms of stress, but it's possible. Coherent breathing is a technique that has an equal length inhale and exhale. To practice, inhale for a count of three or four, and exhale for the same count. Matching the two will balance the nervous system, and the body will feel calm and safe. Your stress resilience will increase, and you will be better able to respond calmly and accordingly after obstacles.

....

23. van der Kolk, *The Body Keeps the Score*, 269.
24. Brown and Gerbarg, *The Healing Power of the Breath*, 9.

DAY 107

Easing out of our yoga practice is not just a way to drag out the time. Gentle transitions are healthy for the body, especially after deep concentration. Moving slowly out of shavasana, the final resting pose, and resisting the urge to jump up and put on my shoes has not come naturally to me. By the time the instructor is guiding us down to our mats, my mind is already halfway out the door, thinking ahead to what I need to do that day.

As a teacher, I observe the pull my students feel to sit up quickly as soon as shavasana ends, to bring their palms together, bow, and get out of there. Yes, we all lead very busy lives, and nearing the completion of a yoga practice often makes it that much harder to stay. However, I have learned that there are no wasted parts of our practice. Everything, from the observation of our breath at the beginning to the final rest and transition out, is essential. Each piece contains insight and opportunity. Each moment, each breath, is a plea for you to stay.

Shavasana begins a necessary step along our path. It is the practice of integration and transitioning gently. We begin with deep inhales and exhales. We make small movements with fingers and toes. We allow time for our body and our nervous system to catch up to our minds. Like in life, we don't need to rush the in-between, and we don't need to let the next activity seep into the one before it. Finish strong. Finish mindfully. Be complete, and only then, move to the next thing.

DAY 108

As we've discussed, yoga recognizes that we have two bodies—a physical body and an energetic body, also called the subtle body. Yoga aims to connect these bodies, or at least become aware that they both exist, so we can better understand the differences and the ramifications of each part of ourselves. Focusing only on the physical misses some of what's happening in the energetic Self and vice versa. The breath is the thread that connects the physical and energetic bodies. The breath is both anatomic *and* energetic. So, when we breathe and hold our focus on the sensation of breath, we are connecting body, mind, and heart, which is a main purpose of yoga. The flow of breath relaxes the physical body. The nervous system regulates, muscles soften, and joints remain open.

In *Pranayama*, Yoganand Michael Carroll and Allison Gemmel Laframboise explain, "When we feel more than we are comfortable feeling, our minds often diminish our experience. One way the mind does this is by tightening the body."[25] The flow of breath allows the body to be in a state of receiving, so we may safely acknowledge emotions instead of pushing them away. The breath allows us to feel, so we don't tighten and lock down our experience. We've all experienced the mind-body connection when it comes to stress. We get tight shoulders, or we catch a cold. The physical body reacts when we don't take care of it emotionally. The more open and allowing we can be in our bodies, the better we can process emotions, even uncomfortable ones, rather than let them create physical problems when unacknowledged.

....

25. Laframboise and Carroll, *Pranayama*, 86–87.

DAY 109

Some life experiences break us open to such a state of vulnerability, and our body's natural reaction is to safeguard and protect. Experiences that cause our hearts to expand with love or break from pain feel too raw and exposed for our rational mind. Walls are built. Vulnerable emotions are shut down. But the body holds the emotion anyway, and not allowing ourselves to feel the emotion means it remains a knot—unable to be processed and unable to be freed. We are not free from an experience until we allow ourselves to feel it. Breath is a way to bring ourselves to presence and feel what is happening in the moment. Breath is a way to acknowledge our emotions rather than shut them down. Feeling is enough. There isn't much to figure out or analyze. There's only feeling and accepting in order for energy to move.

When we allow our walls to come down, we trust ourselves enough to have a full human experience, an experience that includes a range of emotions, rather than a life of safety and limited awareness. Feeling sensations creates opportunities to move through an experience, a relationship, a beginning, or an end. With this new perspective, there is nothing to fear and nothing to close off. In fact, living a life open will bring you more love, more joy, more compassion, and more fulfillment than living with a body that refuses to experience confusing or painful emotions. A life of vulnerability and the capacity to feel allows us to live in the depths rather than the surface. It also means gaining a deep understanding of others, compassion for the human experience, and healing for yourself and the world.

DAY 110

Prana is life force, the sustaining energy that exists in every living thing. Mammals, reptiles, trees, insects, the sea, and the wind—prana is everywhere. Life force floats under a bird's wings and moves the clouds. This same pranic energy flows through our bodies.

One day I spent twenty minutes watching my black lab play with a bumble bee. The fuzzy bee hovered above the dog's nose, tempting her. I waited for the bee's sting and the dog's yelp that never came. The dog bent down and set her chin on the ground, and the bee followed, resting itself on tips of grass, still tickling the dog's nose. They continued. One would go up and the other followed, then down, then side to side. They danced. The dog was curious; the bee was trusting. The dog lifted a paw and attempted to swat. The bee zipped sideways and then came back. The dog wagged her tail in approval. How do a seventy-five-pound dog and a half-inch bee interact? How do they recognize each other's existence, and how can each of their true essences mingle so sweetly with the other's?

Yoga teaches us union and acceptance of Self. Prana teaches that every living thing holds the same life force. To connect with prana, lie in the grass and feel the soft blades under your palms. Sit up against a thick tree and ask an important question. Walk barefoot. Dance in the wind. Stare at the moon. In nature, our bodies forget useless identities and remember that we are energy. When you are present with nature, you might notice what you thought was impossible.

DAY 111

If our life force is the same breath that allows trees to bloom and the sun to rise, then we are connected to the earth and everything on it in more ways than we know. Just like the tree flowers and fades with each season, we can trust that our bodies and our circumstances will do the same. Everything is temporary yet necessary. Everything is in our best interest if we pay attention.

The trick to flowing with life is to keep our prana strong and our mind focused. Both prana and mental energy need to be resolute in order to remain steadfast among the pulls and lures of life. When we get too busy or overwhelmed, we lose focus, and the mind wanders to stories and attachments. Prana joins in, and we become frantic, excitable, or completely depleted. Once again, we should return to awareness and acceptance through breath. Swami Kripalu advises us to "see to the battle of opposing forces going on within."[26]

When we have a practice and stick to it, the mind reacts less to chaos. Prana is maintained without instigating the mind. If life is particularly stressful and it seems like the mind is winning the battle with prana, practice more, practice longer, and practice with more intention. If you can't make it to your yoga mat, take your yoga practice out with you—to the store, on your walk, or during your morning commute. There is always time and space to watch the breath and balance our energies. Welcome in a focused practice of mindfulness to tame your unruly mind.

....
26. Levitt, *Pilgrim of Love*, 158.

DAY 112
Nadi Shodhana (Channel Cleansing Breathing)

While I would never claim yoga to have magical powers, I do call this next pranayama *magic*. The effectiveness of this breath practice *feels* magical because it lightens the load I am carrying instantly and every single time. This breath is called nadi shodhana (channel cleansing breathing). If I could prescribe nadi shodhana to the entire world to do every day, I believe the world would be less angry and less violent. We would all float a little easier. After doing nadi shodhana with my client, an ER doctor, she showed it to a patient experiencing a panic attack. I was so uplifted! The more people who do yoga and share these beneficial practices, the happier and healthier the world will be.

To practice, begin seated. Bend the pointer finger and middle finger of your right hand down, and turn your hand toward your face. Use your thumb to close the right nostril. Inhale up the left nostril, then close it with your ring finger. Open the thumb and exhale out your right nostril. Inhale up the right side and close it with the thumb. Open and exhale left. Inhale left, close, and open and exhale right. Inhale right, close, and open and exhale left. Continue, creating a horseshoe shape of breath.

Practicing nadi shodhana is like releasing the screaming valve on a pressure cooker. It cleanses the nasal passages, calms the mind, relieves stress, and decreases brain fog. If you are experiencing something overwhelming, this exercise helps the mind let go of fear and shift to a clearer perspective. Despite the long and valid list of scientific benefits, the best way to describe this practice is *magic*.

DAY 113

In the Bhagavad Gita, the ancient Sanskrit text that imparts many lessons from yoga, Krishna mentors Arjuna, a young warrior, on the path of yoga in order to reach self-realization. The story takes place on a physical battlefield, representative of the great battle within, and describes eloquently how to be free of suffering. According to the Gita, there are two paths at the time of death—the path to liberation and the path to rebirth. Rebirth means we come back in human form and endure more suffering. Prana is the path to liberation at the time of death and also during life. Prana is our link to the Divine. A verse from the Gita states, "Remembering me at the time of death, close down the doors of the senses and place the mind in the heart. Then, while absorbed in meditation, focus all energy upwards to the head."[27] By cultivating prana and moving energy upward through yoga, meditation, and living according to our personal truth, we are better able to see the truth of all existence and connect with whatever our version is of an energy greater than ourselves. The Gita is a road map to living our dharma, our soul's purpose. When we follow our own heart, we live the path that is meant for us, thus healing past karma and serving the greater good.

Our yoga practice focuses first on the body as a way to tune in to our sensory experience. Through this continued focus on the senses, we gain awareness of prana and awareness of our inner knowing. We are aware of prana in life so we may recognize the truth of our existence at the time of death.

....
27. Easwaran, *The Bhagavad Gita*, 166.

DAY 114

Instead of trying to "master" a pose, try mastering your inner experience, which looks like letting go of your outer appearance and tuning in to what you feel. Do not underestimate the power of permission in a yoga class or in your personal practice. If we only focus on "correct" postures with no room to feel, we miss a valuable part of our practice—the ability to answer our inner calling.

Once during a class, my instructor invited us to bring our body into whatever form it wanted. "Move how it feels *essential*. What does your body *crave?*"

The responsibility of her request made my body freeze up with unsureness. What if I chose wrong? As if reading my mind, the teacher added, "There is no wrong choice."

I wanted to get an A+ in yoga. I wanted to "master" the poses and get it right. I had never considered asking my body what it craves. After an initial lag in my senses, I began moving freely however it felt best. I don't know what I did or what I looked like. At first, I felt silly and awkward, but after a few minutes, I was smiling ear to ear. What freedom! What self-love! What contentment!

My chemical response to permission was so pure and alive during yoga, and I wanted to feel this way—happy, joyous, fulfilled, and true to myself—all the time. If we can move from our breath and our intuition in yoga, then we can also move this way in life. We don't have to worry how others are moving or how we look in comparison. Mastering our inner experience shifts our outside world.

DAY 115

We can easily get caught up in our minds and let our thoughts talk us out of something. We have an idea or a desire, but as soon as the thought arrives, so do a million reasons we can't or we shouldn't. Yes, there are practicalities in life, such as geography, finances, and commitments, and I am not saying we can go about the world with complete abandon and disregard. Things have a way of working themselves out when we lean into what we truly want, though. Money appears, people show up, synchronicities occur, and things fall into place. At the very least, we don't have to immediately disregard every idea that arrives.

Through breath, we can tune in to our desires and allow what is within us to float to the surface of our being. When connected to our breath, we become aware of inner longings and personal truths. We do not have to spend so much time being dragged around by the whims or wants of others—or by our own expectations. We can honor that hobby, passion, career choice, or pastime. We don't have to feel irresponsible or indulgent for living our truth. In fact, it is our highest responsibility to bring our truth forth. The truth will set us free.

You know what lights you up. You know what makes you get out of bed in the morning. Your passion may not make a million dollars, but it's meaningful because it's *yours*. There is a gift within you. Not allowing that gift to come forth cheats you of the experience of feeling truly and unapologetically *you*. Not sharing your gift with the world prevents the world from receiving the reason you are here.

DAY 116

This practice has been all about breath. What have you tried? What have you learned? What new awareness about yourself is now at the surface? If there is a particular pranayama you enjoy, keep doing it. If there is a technique you struggle with, well, you could get curious. I have disliked kapalabhati and the fastness and the pumping of my stomach it requires, which means there is probably a lesson for me there. So, I will keep practicing with gentleness and exploration.

Remember that at the heart of yoga is the breath. Watching the breath, just as it is, is a very powerful practice all on its own. You do not need a fancy technique or complicated mantras in order to meditate and achieve states of pure awareness while watching the breath. Observing the breath brings us to presence and also draws our attention inward to our body, to our heart, and to our deepest longings. Observing the inhale and exhale becomes its own sustaining practice. Can you sit for five minutes? What about ten?

While observing the breath, you might notice subtle shifts in your awareness. Your mind might expand to a different view, and it is okay to allow this. You might notice that you can observe the breath while also observing other parts of yourself. You might hear sounds in the room or notice smells while still holding focus on the breath. Your mind might float somewhere else completely and then come back. Notice the mind cannot attach to story while watching the breath. The mind cannot observe and also create a narrative. After five minutes or so, open your eyes. Where are you? Where have you been? And what new awareness has arrived?

DAY 117
Ha Breath

Stand in tadasana. On an inhale, raise your arms in front of you and up overhead. On the exhale, lower the arms down in front of you and back to your sides. Do this as many times as feels sufficient, moving the arms at the same pace as the breath—inhaling to rise and exhaling to lower. When you feel ready, exhale and bend the knees as you lower your arms, folding the torso forward and letting the arms swing up behind you. Inhale and swing the arms back up, straightening the legs and standing tall with arms extended. The next time you exhale and fold, open your mouth and say, "Ha!" as the arms swing down and behind you, flung by their own weight. Let this movement flow. Flow with the breath. Keep the arms heavy and swinging. Keep the knees soft and bouncing. Let the head dangle as you release, "Ha!"

Be mindful of the movement in this exercise, which can speed up quickly. If you get dizzy, slow down and come back to standing. Allow the breath to return to normal. Otherwise, if your body enjoys the energy, keep going. *Ha* breath releases negativity and cleanses the throat and abdomen. The audible sound when you say or shout "Ha" creates vibration in the body and moves stuck energy. After a few rounds, you may feel lighter—as if something has been let go. Allow yourself to savor the completion of this posture. Standing in mountain pose, watch the dust settle. Observe your breath and your heartbeat. Notice tingling in the limbs. Bring yourself eye-to-eye with the still point, the quiet after the fervor, the settling after the churning.

DAY 118

The simplicity of reminding you to breathe is not meant to minimize your stress, worry, or anything you are going through. When you have a problem, the advice to "take deep breaths" is not a flippant response. The reminder to breathe is because it is the fastest way to remember who we are, where our power lies, and what we can and can't control. The breath, which we often taken for granted, is our life force, our anatomical sustenance that we need to survive. But the breath also controls our emotional body, which, in yoga, is called the subtle body. The subtle body exists beneath the layers of identity, culture, religion, role, status, and personality. The subtle body is our essence, our true Self.

Under normal circumstances, our true Self already battles our ego for attention. Under stress, loss, or illness, the ego gains more power because in these moments, we are vulnerable and fearful. We fear living up to expectations. We fear the unknown. We doubt our own capacity. Breathing through moments of fear, doubt, and the unknown helps us to remember who we are. Through breath, we are immediately connected and tethered to the part of us that knows. Your true Self understands that everything will be okay. Your true Self doesn't need to see the bigger picture to know that it is good. Stop and breathe.

> Inhale and say, "I."
> Exhale and say, "Am."
> *I am. I am. I am.*
> Let that be enough.

DAY 119

We live in a world full of egos with each person fighting for attention, walking around with unhealed wounds, reacting from past hurts, and having no awareness of what they are feeling. It can feel like a mess. We wonder why we do all this work, why we stick to our practice. We wonder if any of it matters. Of course your practice matters. In my experience, egos pull each other around. I have an energetic home with two boys and a dog. They all fight for my attention, often at the same time. If I'm rushed, stressed, or tired, it's easy for my ego to get pulled in by their outbursts. Pretty soon, we are all fighting with each other and with ourselves.

This is when the breath becomes vitally important. It doesn't have to be a home or family situation. You could be at work, running errands, or at the coffee shop. During daily interactions with people, watch your ego try to get your attention. Watch when your ego jumps right in and tries to narrate a situation or encounter. Recognize your ego and how it grasps for control. We can be very calm and centered and, in an instant, be yanked right out of our peaceful state.

The breath reminds us that external chaos need not define our sense of peace. The breath reminds us we always have the power to be still and do nothing. The breath reminds us we cannot control any outcome and any reaction. All of these are true—all of the time and in any situation.

DAY 120

The breath is never forced. The breath flows, and as the witness, we observe. When we do restrain or control the breath, we do so with curiosity and gentleness. We explore the depths and capabilities of the breath but without an intention of grandness or willful manipulation. During any pranayama, we are still the witness. Any technique we practice is out of a desire to get more intimate with our deeper Self, not to prove anything.

Dirgha pranayama is a great way to practice allowing rather than forcing. I describe how to practice dirgha on day 24. Dirgha means "length" and is a three-part yogic breath that begins by inhaling into the belly. Physiologically, when we inhale through the nose, the diaphragm contracts, which allows the belly to expand and the lungs to fill. The body knows how to breathe. Practicing dirgha is a way to observe the breath enter and expand the belly, then the lungs. We don't need to force or push the belly out, and doing so will not increase the benefits.

A way to gain more benefits is by lengthening the inhale and letting our body do the rest. Lengthening the inhale will bring more air in, and the diaphragm will strengthen. The belly will expand as a result of a long breath in. The lungs will fill and the rib cage will expand. Find more breath by lengthening and by taking longer to complete the inhale. Sip air in evenly through your nose. Notice the belly slowly fill and expand. Nothing to force. Nothing to manufacture. By offering space for breath to enter and by allowing rather than forcing, the breath will be nourishing for the body and insightful for the mind.

DAY 121
BRFWA Meditation

For today's practice, try this meditation using BRFWA, Kripalu's signature method meaning breathe, relax, feel, watch, and allow.

Begin seated or in any relaxing position for the body. Close your eyes and begin with a gentle body scan. Observe how the body feels. Then bring your attention to the breath. Observe the breath as it is in this moment. Soften the entire body, and continue to observe the natural sensation of breath, body, heartbeat, surface, weight, and lightness.

Let the breath find a rhythm. You might feel like lengthening the natural inhale and equally lengthening the natural exhale. Do not force the breath. Allow the breath to be easeful. After some moments of easeful breathing, release all control of the breath. Let go of technique and time. Let go of how you think you should breathe or how you think you should meditate. Just let go and watch. Watch where the mind goes. Watch the mind watching the breath or anything happening in the present. Observe what happens. Become the witness of your experience. Watch your mind creating thoughts. Listen to any sounds. Always return to your breath as an anchor. Watch and breathe. Watch and breathe.

When you leave this meditation, you may want to keep your eyes closed or look at the floor. Did you notice a shifting of sensations? Did you notice how energy or thoughts came but then passed through? By allowing all things to be and by staying anchored in the sensation of breath, you were able to have an aware experience—a real experience.

DAY 122

Physically, the breath sustains life and brings our nervous system into balance. Spiritually, the breath helps us with one of the main intentions of yoga—to discern what is true and real. When we breathe deeply and slowly, we are able to listen. The noise of the world and inside ourselves is quieted, so we can hear. Of course between outside circumstance and the mind running wild with stories and thoughts, we are pulled by false beliefs and untrue realities.

What is true? What is real?

These questions are essential to your practice. We spend our lives defining our identity based on what happened to us or what someone said to us. Yoga teaches us that we can discern for ourselves what is true and real. Are you smart? Are you strong?

Yoga is a path of inquiry, which means we ask questions along the way. These are questions about what arrives and questions about how we feel. We open ourselves up to actually listening instead of assuming we already know the answer—instead of assuming someone else knows the answer for us. As a result of our practice, we are at once exposed and empowered.

Now is not the time to abandon yourself. Your practice is opening many possibilities. These are possibilities in who you are and what is true and real today.

PRACTICE 5
Presence (Pratyahara)

Presence is a powerful practice all on its own, and it is also a foundation for reaching deeper stages of awareness. In Patanjali's Eight Limbs, presence is called *pratyahara*, and it precedes meditation and enlightenment.[28] In Hatha yoga, presence is cultivated through breath and movement in order to increase self-awareness. In Kripalu yoga, presence is the first stage in experiencing complete letting go and samadhi (pure being).[29] Simply put, presence is being aware of what is and not being attached to a story from the past or a worry in the future. Being present is experiencing the moment without labels or expectations. Presence is simple but difficult to achieve. Rarely are we free from the mind. Rarely are we present in our actions. Presence is integral to yoga because without presence, we cannot reach other energetic states or grasp an awareness of our deeper Self. Once presence is established, the other stages, such as meditation, freedom, and enlightenment, become possible.

. . . .

28. Satchidananda, *The Yoga Sutras of Patanjali*, 117.
29. *Kripalu School of Yoga Meditation Training Manual*, 14.

DAY 123

The Sanskrit word for "presence" is *pratyahara*, and it is the fifth Limb of Yoga on the Eight-Limbed Path. *Pratyahara* translates to "withdrawal of senses."[30] In our practice, we bring attention to our breath and physical sensations in order to draw the mind inward rather than outside with so many distractions. We can practice presence in our day-to-day by allowing ourselves to be accepting of the current moment. Being present doesn't mean we need to be happy with a situation, but we can allow ourselves to feel it, to be present with it, instead of going down the road of distraction or self-abandonment. We all know our patterns. When I get uncomfortable, I scroll through my phone or shop online instead of being in the moment. I eat something sweet. I can actually watch myself doing these things as a way to cope. Don't beat yourself up. Of course we will reach for distractions when it's too much to sit still, but with awareness of how the mind works, we can be more discerning about our choices and act less on autopilot. By being present with what is, we can accept the situation and possibly learn.

Practicing presence brings contentment and ease to our activities and our spirit. In the next readings, I will discuss the role and benefits of presence on our mat and in our everyday life. In addition to being present with the moment, I will also share practices that leave the confines of presence in order to explore the next stages of spiritual awareness.

....
30. Satchidananda, *The Yoga Sutras of Patanjali*, 117.

DAY 124

The practice of pratyahara is rich with ancient yoga philosophy. The concepts can feel overwhelming and complex, but I find they are very applicable to our modern day. They can help us not only navigate life but also attain peace and ease in a busy, material world. Presence is simple but not easy. Our mind will always try to lure us away—away from the present moment, away from our body, and away from our true Self. Pratyahara is the practice of removing outside senses so we can direct our attention and our efforts inward. Presence is a practice in touching and sensing what is real and right in front of us. When we are present, we are content. Outside problems and struggles do not disappear, but being present allows us to experience relief from the worrying mind.

Consider that the mind is always in the past or in the future. Neither are real right now. Pratyahara allows us to truly glimpse presence, and I say *glimpse* because the experience is often fleeting. It is rare that even a seasoned yogi can experience long moments of complete presence. Our mind is conditioned to continually produce thoughts, which means we are continually asked to notice them and let them pass through. Presence doesn't mean we will ever be free from distraction. Just like meditation does not guarantee we will ever have a completely empty mind. Presence is a practice like anything else. It something we must return to—again and again—as a reminder to bring ourselves back to what is real.

DAY 125

You have already been practicing pratyahara. In addition to a physical exercise, yoga allows us to take a break from what's happening in our day and bring our attention inside. The combination of breath and movement is helpful in quieting the busy mind; it's difficult to focus on what we need to do that day or on a stress or worry when we have a concentrated focus on our breath and our body.

Sometimes, presence happens by accident, and the body is usually involved. Consider a time when you were sad or anxious. Then something made you laugh. Maybe a friend said something funny, or maybe you witnessed a comical interaction. While laughing, even briefly, you were free from your pain. Your mind was not stuck on the thoughts or stories attached to your situation. This scenario demonstrates how the body is able to be present and happy despite an outside circumstance and despite how you feel. Happiness is always available through the present moment. In the present moment, nothing is actually wrong—at least not in the way our mind is telling us. You can also be present with negative emotions. Presence grants access to a real experience. Nothing more and nothing less.

DAY 126
Vrikshasana (Tree Pose)

Begin standing. Find your foundation and your strength in tadasana. Feel both feet evenly on the earth. Find a drishti, or a visual spot to keep focus, such as a spot on the floor or somewhere in front of you. Then shift your weight into your left leg and foot. Observe this shift, and with your toes on the mat, open your right knee to the right. Check that your hips stay square to the front rather than following the knee and also opening. You may feel sensation in your right hip. Stay here in tree pose. If you choose, place the sole of your foot on your ankle or calf. Now find length. Press down through the standing left foot and use the support of the earth to get taller and lengthen through the crown of your head. Remember to breathe. If you tip or wobble, observe the body and its muscles gently. Watch if the mind is generating thoughts and criticisms and come back to the body.

Determine where you can exert more effort, and where you can exert less. Breathe. Find length. Feel the standing leg, energy through the spine, arms floating upward but not grasping.

A balance like tree pose is a great way to practice presence. Balance postures require a drishti, a single focus for our sight. Balance poses also require concentration and an examination of effort and ease in the body. When the mind gets involved, we can return to the breath, a great way to practice staying present. If you fall, come back. Falling out of balance and returning is a powerful learning experience for the body and the mind.

DAY 127

Let's explore an explanation of presence from the Sutras. Although I have been talking a lot about getting out of the mind in order to access presence and truth, the mind is not the enemy. The Sutras refer to the mind as "mind-stuff," meaning the mind behaves a certain way but the thoughts are just that—*stuff*—and not necessarily truth.[31] Many disturbances in the mind are caused by outside stimuli and our perception of them but not the mind itself. There are stimuli all around us—media, people, opinions, information, noise. The trick to staying centered and true to who you are is to remove the mind from its associations with outside objects. It is impossible to view anything in our outside world without attaching a belief or opinion. Even if we experience something as basic as a table, it has the ability to insight memory. Even recognizing the object as a table takes perception. Often, we are ruled by the outside. As stimuli come in, the mind attaches, and we view according to our perception.

In contrast, through focused concentration on breath and sensations, we can draw the mind inward so it is not as bothered by outside perception. Senses are neutral in the mind. Therefore, when the mind is turned inward, when senses take on the quality of mind as the witness, the mind is at peace. According to Patanjali's Sutras, "When the senses withdraw themselves from the objects and imitate, as it were, the nature of the mind-stuff, this is Pratyahara."[32] Witness how the mind works and attaches, and you will be practicing presence.

....

31. Satchidananda, *The Yoga Sutras of Patanjali*, 155.
32. Satchidananda, *The Yoga Sutras of Patanjali*, 155.

DAY 128

According to Patanjali and many practicing yogis, we can actually master the senses and then master the mind. I am definitely not there, but it is an inspiring concept. By changing our reaction to the senses, by mastering our ability to recognize a sense as simply that—a sensation—we attain freedom from the belief that attaching to a desire will bring fulfillment. Consider eating a delicious meal. Our senses tell us we will experience joy at the first smell of brownies cooking. We eat the brownie, and it tastes delicious in our mouth and on our tongue. Soon, our experience changes, and we might feel an ache in our belly as our body starts to digest the sweet indulgence. We realize our senses are not always accurate. At the least, they continually change and shift. Yoga does not tell us we should avoid life's pleasures. In fact, we can eat the brownie, enjoy a delicious meal, and respond to our desires. But we forgo the expectation that any joy experienced from an outside indulgence will be permanent. Once we have this awareness, we have developed some mastery. We will stop mindlessly reaching for something or someone to complete us. We will be able to enjoy simple pleasures without craving more or longing for a different experience. With mastery of the senses, we are no longer bound by outside circumstance. Instead, we are grounded in the truth that real satisfaction comes from within and understanding of the fact that to experience freedom, we must free ourselves from the belief that external pleasure results in permanent peace.

DAY 129

Presence helps us master our senses and our experience. Presence does not promise to get rid of the inner workings of the mind, but it helps us to be at peace with what is. Once we realize the mind is not always reliable and that it will always produce thoughts and perceptions, we have more control over our experience.

Through awareness and acceptance, yoga lovingly heals everything we have been too afraid to look at, even wounds we didn't realize were there. Yoga brings into question the belief that we are not good enough, not deserving, or not capable. Yoga takes us away from comparison, inner critique, and self-doubt and shows us we are strong, worthy, and a being of light. With a yoga practice centered in ethical behaviors, we discover the gift of nonviolent living and pure intention. We improve our own character, so we can more gracefully interact with others. We become better humans, so we can serve humanity. Yoga does not ask us to prove anything or be anything. Presence is a practice in observing, not denying or berating. The Eight Limbs and other texts share practices and potential effects, but yoga is not an assignment or a test. Yoga is not an exact image or precise chain of events. Yoga is personal. Every experience and every pain point are paramount to your yoga practice. Every part of you is relevant and essential. Presence and awareness of the mind is a start. The poses and the breath are a way in. By practicing presence, by noticing the behaviors and tendencies of the mind, we are staying present with what is, and we are less affected by the outside world.

DAY 130

As much as we want to manage, fix, and change everything in our outside world, the real change happens when we look within. It's very challenging to not let things bother us, especially when we care. Being present does not mean we stop caring. We still have reactions to people, places, and things. Of course we will get angry or frustrated, sad or hopeless, but at our core, at the center of who we are, we are not pulled away from ourselves. There is a big difference between having a reaction to something that bothers or hurts us and believing something different about ourselves as a result of the situation. Not getting the promotion does not mean we are bad at our job. Being betrayed in our relationship does not mean we did anything to cause it. It's always helpful to look at our role in situations in order to grow and improve, but we don't need to pile on more responsibility than is ours to carry. We don't have let the experience, good or bad, define who we are. Who we are is constant and unshakable.

There are going to be life events that change and shape us. Loved ones die, relationships end, we endure illness and the unthinkable. The most painful moments, if we can stay present, teach us so much. One of the greatest lessons I have learned from yoga is how to stay. How to look something in the face and not run. How to dig into the unshakable part of myself and, as much as it hurts, trust myself enough to endure. We are stronger when we come out the other side. We are wiser because we did not run away from the present.

DAY 131

At first, we might be surprised to notice how often we are not present. It's possible you thought you were present most of the time, but once you start observing presence with more intention, you realize how much you are in story—story about the past or worry about the future. Awareness is the first step. We all stumble out of presence, but with awareness, we can learn to come back more quickly.

To practice presence, we do not necessarily need to eliminate outside distraction. In fact, this is unrealistic. We will always have jobs to complete, people to care for, and desires and passions that keep us in the outer experience. We want to be human and ride with the ups and downs of life, but we don't want to be at the mercy of outside circumstance to the point that we lose sight of who we are. It helps to notice when we are *not* present and understand the consequences of this.

For example, this week I allowed myself to be pulled away several times, and it caused unnecessary stress. Instead of focusing on myself and what I needed to accomplish, such as writing, an upcoming course, and taking care of myself, I became obsessed with other people and distractions. I was on social media way too much. I became anxious and lashed out at a friend. I fed my fear and remained *unpresent*. And the result was my own suffering. If you're acting in a way that makes you feel anxious or bad, you're probably not present. If you're resisting presence by focusing on other people and tasks instead of yourself, notice. Ask why. Fear from feeling something can keep us from presence.

DAY 132

Just like a drishti helps us stay balanced in a pose, a single-pointed focus during yoga or meditation is useful in order to stay present. The mind likes to wander, and as committed as we are to our practice, intention alone doesn't always keep us tuned in. It can be helpful to have a focus, such as the breath or mantra. This is why we start each yoga practice by bringing attention to the breath. After a few breaths, our mind naturally lets go, and thoughts no longer feel so important or alluring. In this moment, there is the breath. In this moment, we can watch the inhale and the exhale. In this moment, there is nothing else to do and no one else to be.

Another way to stay tethered to the moment is with the use of mantra. The Sanskrit word for this is *japa*. A japa or intention can be repeated, either out loud or in your mind, as a way to stay focused. If there is a phrase you like, use it. Japa does not need to be some ancient poem or prayer, although it certainly can be. One of my favorite ways to meditate is to settle in for a few breaths, ask my inner Self what I need, and let a word or phrase arrive. Say your japa out loud. Then continue repeating the words to yourself. When your word or phrase starts to feel forced, let it go. Loosen your attachment to the words themselves, and let their energy expand throughout your body and senses. Sit with the mantra. When it feels complete, release it.

DAY 133

I like to think of presence as a practice to manage outside distractions, such as when a child or a pet interrupts your yoga practice. Distractions can also be internal, such as when a worry or obsessive thought won't leave your mind. Any distraction, external or internal, can prevent us from being present or in a meditative state.

We all have experienced the peace and inspiration after a *perfectly undisturbed* yoga session. All is quiet, both in our home and in our mind, and we flow easily through the poses. We connect to the breath, and at the end of our practice, we feel rejuvenated and at peace. There are also those times when our yoga practice does not feel so peaceful or easy. There is noise. There are people or circumstances that threaten to pull us away. Someone needs us. We resist our mat and wonder if we are being selfish by taking this time. We rush through poses. We wonder when it will end. We skip the ending, and we walk away from our mat frustrated, still disturbed.

During any yoga or meditation practice, we can be accepting and forgiving. We can accept distraction, inside and out, and know that every practice will not meet our rigid expectations. When we accept that our practice and our life might not always go as planned, we keep our power. Pratyahara asks us to act in alignment with ourselves, which means noticing when we show up despite everything that threatens to take us away. Practicing yoga in a quiet, undisturbed environment is easy. Practicing yoga in life, which often contains many distractions, is the true practice.

DAY 134

Sometimes, everything can be going so well, and all of a sudden, your body is thrown into a state of anxiety or unease. Discerningly, you look around. Nothing is out of place. Nothing is wrong. Yet, in your body, something feels amiss.

During moments of anxiety, cultivating the witness is an excellent tool. Witness consciousness is the part of us that can observe the present moment without distraction, without a story. Yogis call this "pure awareness," and it is when we can alternate between the mind that is in thought and the mind that is the witness. In the Sutras, *nirodha parinama* is the conjunction of thought and one's effort to restrain or modify it.[33] Cultivating the witness is not to rid the mind of thought but to become aware of the mind's workings. A few practices that can help cultivate witness consciousness are yoga, moving the body, or meditation. We can also go for a walk and observe nature. We can activate all our senses. What do we see, feel, hear, taste, and smell? When we learn that our mind will take us to places that are not present, we can gently and compassionately discern between real threat and the mind's trickiness. We can kindly pull ourselves out of a panic attack by relying on the present to point us to truth.

When you start to feel anxious, bring your senses to the present. Become the witness. Observe your body and your surroundings. It becomes empowering to watch the two minds—the mind that's all over and the mind that's the witness—observe things just as they are.

....

33. Satchidananda, *The Yoga Sutras of Patanjali*, 168.

DAY 135

There are many myths about meditation. These include what to do, how to sit, and what it should feel like. Meditation is a state of mind, one where we are fully present and fully able to experience the current moment. Rather than think of meditation as something you do, like a technique, think of meditation as something you are as a result of presence. By practicing presence, you arrive in a new awareness, and this loving awareness is meditation.

Meditation is a sustained amount of time in the present. I have entered states of meditation while journaling, walking, and cleaning. We can be present while doing activities that bring us out of the rational mind and into a more relaxed state of awareness. Meditation feels like clarity. I would also describe it as a feeling of oneness, like everything is connected and everything will be okay. I am completely at ease. I am full of love. I have no regrets and no judgment. For me, meditation happens briefly. If I am doing yoga, focused on breath and movement, I can be in meditation longer.

To meditate, get present. Be in a comfortable seated position or lie down. You can also be walking mindfully. Once present, find a focus. Observe the breath, a cloud, or a sound. Stay connected to the senses rather than thoughts. Allow your awareness to expand, and see if you sense anything different—anything that feels like love or deeper awareness of your true nature and the true purpose of meditation.

DAY 136

According to neuroscience, we are not the same person from one day to the next. In *Awakening the Brain*, Charlotte Tomaino writes, "Our brains change with every experience … We are evolving in every moment with the chemistry of each sound, sight, thought, and emotion that passes through the brain."[34] Neuroplasticity is the brain's ability to create new neuropathways—new reactions to experience—based on our choices. Tomaino writes that making new choices changes our experience and therefore changes our brain.[35] Neuroplasticity helps to explain how meditation works to change the brain. When we sit and observe the senses, when we take ourselves out of story and routine reactions, we are better able to discern our real experience from an old pattern. Through presence and meditation, we can train the brain to perceive experiences differently.

Let's say you have a negative reaction to a particular person. Your interaction leaves you anxious, and you don't know why. You may even anticipate your reaction. This is how conditioned and automatic your reaction is. Just like how we remember to ride a bike, the brain remembers our experiences. Once we reframe our brain and choose new reactions, we start to remove and replace old conditioning. Next time you encounter this person, arrive with openness and compassion. Know that you don't have to react the same way you always have. Make a different choice, and see if it changes your present reality.

....

34. Tomaino, *Awakening the Brain*, 33.
35. Tomaino, *Awakening the Brain*, 34.

DAY 137

We are not bound by our habits, patterns, or routines. Just like in a yoga pose, we always have the choice to stay, try something new, or back out. We make this choice by observing the sensations in our body and determining what is best for us in that moment. We understand that this moment is crucial. Tomorrow's practice or yesterday's practice has nothing to do with the choice we make for ourselves today. It is one thing to have a schedule and a discipline; however, once inside the practice, we can lend ourselves grace to act differently. If we are always trying to make our current practice look the same as another, we miss the opportunity to practice what is needed for ourselves in the present moment.

This is the case for life too. We might not need the same exact routine one morning as we did the day before. We might not need the same meal, the same social situations, or the same self-care. Enacting presence does not look the same moment to moment. Enacting presence means we are flexible enough to actually listen to our needs. Our mind can easily "think" we need something when, in fact, we are operating on past patterns. We may not even be hungry at noon, but we eat anyway because that's what we're used to. Only when we are open, only when we are truly engaged in the practice of presence, are we able to make choices based on current circumstance rather than habit and automation. Let go of what happened yesterday. The present moment is rich with opportunity, and there is no way to get it wrong other than to stop listening.

DAY 138

What do you reach for when you feel an uncomfortable emotion or when something is pulling you away from the present moment? When you worry, do you rush to find a solution, or do you look for a way to escape? Both choices might be ignoring what is happening in the present moment. Both decisions might take us away from what our body needs in order to actually address the worry or problem.

When we are doing too much, we are not present. When we are lazy, apathetic, and hopeless, we are not present. Each of us can easily rush through life and not pay attention to the stress that is building. We can also give up and spend a weekend on the couch, eating ice cream, or doing anything else that helps us forget.

Neither of these reactions to stress is bad. Being lazy and being active can both be necessary forms of self-care when done in small amounts and when we are aware. We may tend toward one of the two routes to avoid stress, either overdoing or underdoing. Some of us avoid by isolating and being lazy. Some of us avoid by adding tasks and overworking. To practice yoga is to enact the witness. It is to observe if we are in balance or if we are swinging too far in either direction.

In reaction to anything stressful in your life right now, what can you do in order to achieve more balance? Some options are meditation, yoga, walking, being in nature, a hobby you enjoy, or spending time with a person you care about. Be aware and intentional, observing lovingly what your tendency is and how you might guide yourself back to center.

DAY 139

Our practice never ends. There is never a moment when we will have everything figured out and be able to say, "*I no longer need my practice.*" This is why we return, again and again. We return to remember who we are. We return because each time we taste the sweetness of acceptance and a feeling of love for ourselves and others, like a yummy dessert, we want to taste it again and again. We return because it is human nature to forget. We return because glimpsing the soul is just that—a glimpse. For a moment during meditation, a deep shavasana, or as we hold balancing half moon for the first time, we might glimpse that we are actually loved, actually worthy, and actually capable of more than we know. We might allow our bodies to feel and to cry. We might forgive ourselves or someone else, freeing ourselves from the heaviness of our past. We might journey somewhere inside ourselves we were once too afraid to enter. We might uncover pain but along with it an eerie sense that the love is abundant, overflowing, and pure.

We return to our practice because the insight we receive is always helpful to our life. Another day, another problem, and another moment of self-doubt will always arrive. We practice on the days we feel good, so we will remember who we are on the days we feel bad. We return because of the promise from the Sutras. It is the promise that says our practice is not only for our own peace but for others because "with a peaceful mind, you can go out into the world and serve well."[36]

....
36. Satchidananda, *The Yoga Sutras of Patanjali*, 26.

DAY 140

I started meditating when I didn't know what was wrong and didn't know what to do. I was unable to feel any emotions other than anger, resentment, and fear. The critical voice in my head was the only voice I heard. I literally felt crazy, and I had read that meditation could change my brain. Maybe if I could heal my brain, I wouldn't feel so terrible all the time.

I started each morning by sitting in an old chair I had salvaged from the side of the road and recovered in shaggy white fabric. I set a timer on my phone for ten minutes, crossed my ankles beneath me, and closed my eyes. I didn't move until my phone rang the peaceful chimes. I had no idea what I was doing. I only knew that if I could stick to this routine, something in my soul and my life might improve. I did this nearly daily for a year. On the days I skipped, my mood was different, more impatient, more likely to spiral into depressing thoughts and unhealthy behaviors. Part of me knew how to meditate, and that same part of me knew I needed it. Despite not having a guide or a template, I knew how important these ten minutes were. The meditation was not perfect; I may not have done anything according to technique. But that is not the point of meditation. The point is to show up. Even if I spent the entire ten minutes lost in my thoughts or checking off to-do lists, something small shifted. After a year, I was a different person. Show up and the practice works on you.

DAY 141

I taught English as a second language for eighteen years. While the curriculum focused on language, grammar, writing, and pronunciation, much of the class was also dedicated to assimilation, to understanding a culture and becoming aware of behaviors and customs. Things a native speaker takes for granted. Learning a second language is conscious at first. We locate the words, string together the proper grammar, and intentionally form the syllables to speak. After much practice, the language embeds into our subconscious. We don't need as much rational thought to communicate.

Preceding my career in ESL, I studied abroad in Spain my junior year of college. Even though I had taken many years of Spanish, when I showed up in the country, I felt like I had learned nothing. After two weeks of bumbling through conversations and feeling like a failure, I went from understanding nothing to understanding everything. It was as if part of my brain shifted over. I went from analyzing every word to feeling the language flow out of me. My body simply needed to experience all the smells, tastes, sounds, touches, and sights of this new place. The foreign needed to become familiar in every single sense, not just the grammar I had learned in the classroom. The mind is rational; the body is sensory. Both are necessary to navigate our experience. To practice presence is to become familiar with how our body responds to experience as much as the mind does. To embody is to feel with all senses. The more we observe our experience, the more we access our subconscious, and we don't have to "think" so much about what we are feeling. Feeling fully becomes our natural way of moving through life.

DAY 142

During meditation, we are activating *chitta* and prana. Prana is our breath; chitta is the mind. Prana is our intuition; chitta is our focused attention. Prana moves us to emotion; chitta makes sense of our experience. When prana is strong, we can access deeper levels of awareness. When chitta is strong, we can stay there—present in the awareness.

Prana and chitta work together and help each other out. During a meditation practice, we benefit from cultivating both prana and chitta. Begin with a focus (this is chitta at work). Your focus can be the breath, a mantra, or a sensation. When a thought arrives, or if the mind is particularly active that day, notice. Chitta can discern the active mind and bring us back to our focus. Chitta is aware of thoughts without attaching story. We watch thoughts arrive, and they pass by. We can strengthen chitta and train the mind to observe thoughts without reacting. Only with the focused and discerning awareness of chitta are we able to experience the expanded awareness of prana. After some moments of focused attention, observe prana begin to grow. Notice if emotions or subtle sensations are showing up. Allow for your intuition to be present. Listen with your heart. As prana grows, let yourself follow it. Keep the awareness of your mind while letting other parts of yourself experience the depths and knowing of prana. Watch for both chitta and prana during your self-observation practice. You will become more aware of the existence of each and how they operate and make you feel. Your meditation will become deeper as a result of strengthening these energies.

DAY 143

In Kripalu yoga, there are three stages to meditation: presence, sustained focus, and letting go of will. You can practice all three stages and notice the subtle distinctions of each. Presence is when we arrive on our mat, in our chair, or standing with feet on solid earth. We begin by bringing ourselves right here—to what we sense and feel in this moment, whether that be our seat on a surface, feet on the ground, or breath moving in our torso. Sustained focus is keeping the mind in the present. We are aware of thoughts but not wandering away. We are holding our attention right here—on the breath. After some willful practice, of pulling the mind back to the breath, of returning to the sensation of the surface beneath us, we can enter the third and final stage of meditation. We can let go of willful practice and technique and watch what happens. Letting go enacts an amount of trust in ourselves and the process. Letting go brings us in touch with the subconscious parts of ourselves and allows prana to grow. Our intuition becomes stronger, and we might sense inner longings or deeper clarity. We might rest in ease and feel less forced effort. Often, we want to remain in stages one and two, unwilling to let go and leave the effort behind. We fear that by letting go, we will lose our focus and lose control of the mind. If you slip into daydreaming, allow this to be. If you enter a state of resistance, wondering if you are doing it right, take a breath and let go again. Explore stage three as a new awareness. There is unlimited possibility in what arrives when we let go.

DAY 144

Learning to be still is a gift. There are many ways to escape the present moment: vacations, jobs, family, and friends. Sometimes, the journey we need is the travel into ourselves. Endless possibilities and great wisdom exist within us. Uncovering layers of Self in order to heal brings freedom and enlightenment. When present with what is, exactly as it is, we give attention to energy that may have gotten stuck due to escaping our emotions or not knowing how to deal with intense situations. Rather than tune in, we may have run to something else, an activity or shiny new adventure. We may have sought relief from something outside ourselves, which provided a quick but temporary fix. In order for emotional energy to move, it first needs to be acknowledged. Do not get hung up on exactly what needs to heal and what needs to move. Your body knows and will do this naturally. Sometimes, we are aware of an old wound or pain point, and we sense an unlocking during our practice. There is no need to micromanage the process. Remember to note all experience in the body as sensation rather than narrative. For example, we can feel tightness somewhere in the body and then a lighter sensation as it opens. Embrace what arrives during presence and practice being still with it all. What is moved and released while present will allow you to walk forward healthier, clearer, and more open than before. There will be no need to escape via outside routes because the trapped energy within has been dealt with.

DAY 145

Leave rigidness and explore openness. There is so much to explore in the body and with the breath! The body is rich with opposing sensations, contradictions, unruly emotions, and creative story-telling. When we allow for a full experience, we leave behind the expectation of everything needing to fit into a defined box. We get more comfortable with the unknown and more accepting of the dualities of our existence. We can at once feel joyful and sad-dened. We can experience appreciation for where we are while also longing for something to be different. We can feel nostalgia for something that has ended without needing to go back. Allow-ing for all emotions, sensations, and yearnings means we are being honest with what is. Emotions don't always require a reaction. We can miss someone but be glad we are no longer around them. We can second-guess our choices but stay true to the reasons we made them. A lot of the time we confuse ourselves by thinking we should always be happy or at ease. If not, we believe something is amiss, and we must do something about it. This adds more struggle to a situation than is necessary. Sometimes, emotions simply are. The range we experience means we are human and accepting all parts of ourselves. By observing opposing emotions and letting them be, we get more skilled at noticing how things are instead of how we think they should look or feel. We are more accepting and less reactive. We are able to be at peace with what is—with nothing to do and nothing to change.

DAY 146
Observing Opposite Sides

Stand in tadasana. Observe the right foot, then the left. Shift your weight, pressing down on one foot and then the other. Spend some time rocking back and forth, shifting your weight. Next, feel both feet equally on the earth. Move your awareness up your body. Observe the right side of the body, then the left. Move back and forth, then observe both sides at the same time. Stand firmly in tadasana and observe the entire body—the body as a complete unit.

Noticing the right and left sides of the body integrates the right and left hemispheres of the brain. Each side processes information differently, the right hemisphere recalling experience more visually and the left side acting more linear. When integrated, it's like getting the brain on the same page, and we have clearer understanding, a more accurate experience. You can practice observing one side of the body or one ear, one hand, one eye, and so on in many postures.

From a therapy standpoint, integrating the right and left sides of the brain helps to fully process our experiences. In yoga, we bring attention to one side of the body, then the other in order to observe differences in each side and to activate both hemispheres of the brain. Through comparison, we become aware that one hip is tighter than the other. We observe that a pose does not feel the same on the right side as it does on the left. We learn about the body, and we learn about ourselves. Possibly, we teach the brain a little something about how to fully process an experience. We learn how both hemispheres—and their unique views—are necessary.

DAY 147

Seeing clearly means experiencing reality, not necessarily what is pleasant. Deep in my addiction days, I was delusional. Not only about my addiction but about everyone and even the world around me. Like most addicts, I feared pain. I would make myself believe anything just to remain happy, optimistic, and pleasant. I kept uncomfortable realities at a distance, not having any interest in the larger problems of society. I certainly did not want to look at my part in all of it.

The best gift I have received from my yoga practice is the ability to be compassionate and to see a real experience instead of how I want something to be. Feeling compassion isn't always comfortable. Seeing clearly allows me to see the good, the terrible, and everything in between. The truth of our world can be heartbreaking. The human experience is one of violence, abuse, poverty, and suffering. Of course there is also joy, compassion, kindness, selflessness, and deep love. All of these experiences exist—in some form—in each of our lives. How do we allow ourselves to experience the whole mess of emotions?

People in pain hurt other people. It's overwhelming to think about changing the world. It's overwhelming to think about changing one single person. Guess what's not overwhelming? Changing yourself. Healing yourself. Looking at yourself. Healing means unburdening ourselves from our individual experiences so that we stop hurting others as a result. Healing yourself ripples out into every relationship you have. Healing means we see clearly all the realities of our world. We have the courage and compassion to heal ourselves so that we may operate with a level of compassion that everyone deserves.

DAY 148
Beginning Meditation Practice

Meditation has the myth of being complex and grandiose. The expectation to experience something earth-shattering during each meditation can prevent us from experiencing the simplicity of noticing sensations. Here is a beginning to a meditation practice, which simply asks you to notice your body in this moment.

Close your eyes and begin with a body scan. Notice your feet and where they touch the floor. Notice your seat and where it touches the chair or surface. What do these surfaces feel like? What parts of your skin are touching other parts of clothing or other skin? Can you notice?

Check in if you are pushing yourself to find something deeper. *Is it really significant to simply notice your feet on the floor? Who cares?* Actually, observing our feet on the ground is very significant. Observing our hands in our lap is also significant. These observations are significant because they are truthful and real. Noticing the body brings awareness and acknowledgment of oneself, like an act of love.

The point of sensory meditation is to first notice the body so we may eventually access deeper stages of awareness. I've had revelatory insights during meditation, but most of the time, meditation is uneventful. I sit. I stay. And when finished, I go on with my day. The questions to ask are never: *What happened? What was the big answer?* The question to ask is: *Did I stay with my experience?* Whether that experience was dramatic, simple, profound, or frustrating, the significance is that you were there.

DAY 149

In Sankhya yoga philosophy, there are three ropes, called the three gunas, that tie us to our earthly experience. The three gunas are rajas (fiery energy and doing), tamas (lazy energy and lethargy), and sattva (light and balance). Ideally, we will be in a state of sattva and at ease, without swinging to the other extremes.

In life, it is easy to swing from highs to lows. We get stuck in exhilaration and then despair. We resist the steadiness of the middle road. The simple meditation of observing the body just as it is and not seeking something extravagant or grandiose is an excellent practice in learning the gift of ease. Reaching for extremes might provide a temporary rush, but they are never fully satisfying.

Being really up or really down creates high sensation, but it is not the kind of sensation that brings us a feeling of ease. With practice, ease has become my favorite state. Ease is a place where I can notice the present because I am not up *or* down. I am not lost in excessive sensation. I am right here, present and observing. Rather than swinging from highs and lows, I now seek to be steady. I know the middle road is reliable. I know steady will remain. I know if I can observe what is really happening—the simple, the real, and the tangible, such as my feet touching the floor—then I can stay out of my head and in the moment. Of the three gunas, sattva is the rope we want to stay tied to. It is the rope that provides balance, ease, and light. Presence brings us to sattva. It takes us away from story and away from excess to right here—in truth.

DAY 150

Kriya means "in action" or "in practice." Patanjali emphasizes the importance of kriya yoga—yoga in practice—rather than too much time in study. Through practice, we can minimize the five obstacles to reaching samadhi, or enlightenment. According to the Sutras, the five obstacles are "ignorance, egoism, attachment, hatred, and clinging to bodily life."[37] It's great to study yoga scriptures and learn as much as we can, but the real lessons from yoga come from our practice, on the mat and in life.

Ignorance refers to forgetting oneself, forgetting our divinity, or believing the impermanent is permanent. Egoism is identifying with our ego instead of our soul, or our source. Attachment is relying on pleasure, addiction, and other dependencies. Hatred refers to aversion, aversion to pain, having self-doubt and self-loathing, and remaining separate. Clinging to bodily life refers to fear of death or staying in illusion regarding our true nature.

Can you relate to any or all of these obstacles? Where do they show up in your yoga practice or in your life? Through kriya yoga, through action and practice, we can slowly recognize our ego, our attachments, and our aversions. We can spend time in postures and in relationships in order to observe how the five obstacles play out in our experience. Most inspiring is that when we become aware of an obstacle, we might also become aware of how to remove it.

....
37. Satchidananda, *The Yoga Sutras of Patanjali*, 80.

DAY 151

I've always felt pulled by the obligation to be okay. I have no idea where I learned this. Maybe it's based on the reaction of others. Or maybe I am so uncomfortable with my own emotions, I refuse to let myself go there. For most of my life, I adopted the mantra *Stay pleasant, keep smiling. You are fine.* A friend told me recently that her therapist had given her the challenge of responding to the question "How are you?" with any phrase other than "I'm fine." Her therapist told her we respond so quickly and blindly with *"I'm fine,"* even when that's not what we are at all.

"How are you?"

"I'm fine."

My friend and I agreed we both do this so mindlessly. I couldn't even come up with an alternate response. I'm ... tired. I'm excellent. I'm proud. I'm lonely.

The words feel strange even coming off my tongue. To actually *admit* something? To be clear about how I *really* feel? Whether we respond to another person or admit it to ourselves, acknowledging how we are is a powerful practice. Knowing how we feel and voicing it takes awareness and acceptance. I have learned that trying to be "fine," even when I am not, prevents me from moving through any emotion. I want to be truthful in my words to myself. I want to listen to my heart and give it the care it deserves rather than dismissing everything that arrives for the insignificant sake of "I'm fine."

DAY 152

Silence is a powerful yoga practice and one that brings us face-to-face with presence. Without talking, we are better able to listen. At first, the mind will be very noisy. Free from our own speech, we will come to notice just how much our mind chatters away. All the thoughts moving through may be alarming. The thoughts may be critical or dark. We might feel like this isn't even us—as if the mind must be someone else's—because we would never have these strange thoughts. Silence is said to be a practice for the masters because in silence, we see, hear, and learn so much. We truly get the experience of self-observation by removing our ability to drown ourselves out with spoken words. A day or even a morning spent in silence will lead you to valuable introspection. Issues will become apparent. You will be able to clearly see your strengths, weaknesses, fears, and longings.

Equipped with a loving attitude of nonjudgment, enter a brief period of silence. You'll learn a lot about yourself in a very short amount of time. Your time spent in silence will not only provide helpful insight into how you think and how you want to change, but it will also grant you a closer connection to your practice. By engaging in silence, you will be less resistant to moving inward during practice and less afraid of presence.

DAY 153

It's silly to think of being fearful of the moment. But we all are. The mind gives us space to wander backward or project ahead. It gives us information and perception and tells us how to view something. Can we ever be truly present? For moments, I believe we can. Eckhart Tolle paints a beautiful description of what it's like to practice presence: "Have you listened, truly listened, to the sound of a mountain stream in the forest? Or to the song of a blackbird at dusk on a quiet summer evening? To be aware of such things, the mind needs to be still. You have to put down for a moment your personal baggage of problems, of past and future, as well as all your knowledge; otherwise, you will see but not see, hear but not hear."[38]

We can spend our entire lives lost in nostalgic memories from the past or in wishful fantasies about the future. We can enact judgment and label every situation as good, bad, right, or wrong, clouding reality and feeding the ego. Or we can get still. We can set everything down and observe.

We've practiced presence in many ways—through self-observation, the body, movement, meditation, and silence. We practice presence so it starts to feel more natural and less boring. We get more comfortable not having a label or agenda. We crave being in the moment. We learn the power of witnessing instead of analyzing and the love that arrives when we watch something in nature or answer our own heart. With each quietly observed breath, we experience a moment of presence.

....
38. Tolle, *The Power of Now*, 80.

ƤRACTICE 6
Rewriting Stories (Samskara)

Our beliefs about ourselves and the world and the stories we tell ourselves, whether conscious or unconscious, create our reality. Many stories are so embedded, so subconscious, we treat them as truth. Every experience you have ever had from the time you were born creates a reaction. This reaction forms a belief and, therefore, an imprint. We learn what elicits approval and what does not. We learn how to protect ourselves from pain. We learn how to receive love and affection. We form beliefs about ourselves and our capacities. *Samskara* means "mental imprint" and is used in yoga to explain how our past affects our present circumstance and our beliefs about ourselves and the world. To explore our samskaras, we will look at our stories and use yoga as a path of inquiry. We will get curious. We will ask questions. We will remain open instead of opinionated. Ultimately, we will ask ourselves if these stories are true.

DAY 154

Your practice now is to cultivate what Shunryū Suzuki calls the beginner's mind. As he wrote in *Zen Mind, Beginner's Mind*, "In the beginner's mind there are many possibilities, but in the expert's there are few."[39] Try to let go of thinking you know anything. It sounds weird, but the more you open your mind to new thoughts and ideas, the more possibilities will flow into your awareness. With an open mind and endless options, you'll wonder why you were so tied to your old story.

We're tied to our stories because they are more than just thoughts; they are imprints in our psyche. Every time you do something, there's a residue that you carry into the next experience. Yoga calls these imprints samskaras. These are the scars carried over into our next experience, the wounds that dictate our reality, until we heal the samskara. Samskaras form as a result of a behavior and a reaction—a cause and effect. Something happens to us, and we either shut down or remain open. Something is painful, and we don't like the feeling, so we create a story that will protect us from experiencing that pain again. We build walls and draw conclusions about ourselves or others. Samskaras are emotional scars. And while they might have served us in the past, they deserve to be reconsidered. What is true now? What is real today?

Just like the belief was formed in response to a reaction, when we adopt new behaviors, new reactions to our experience, we rewrite the story. Illuminating samskaras and rewriting stories is a powerful, life-changing practice. Be open. Be a beginner. Today is a new day.

....
39. Suzuki, *Zen Mind, Beginner's Mind*, 1.

DAY 155

Letting go is a great intention, but it requires some focused awareness on patterns and behaviors that contribute to the wound. When we make a choice to let something go, we are also healing a samskara, the psychological groove formed from a particularly memorable experience, that dictates our beliefs and behaviors. Samskaras are healed when we choose a different pattern, and at first, this choice feels very odd, even wrong.

Consider patterned behaviors, such as the way you talk with your partner or parents, the way you react to a person or event, or the way an addiction of any kind takes hold over your cells and your thoughts. All of these patterned behaviors form imprints, which are reinforced with every conditioned reaction. When a samskara is reinforced, we deepen the groove. We add to the pattern, even if it is negative, unhealthy, or not true. We can spend our entire lives stuck in a samskara and never know any different. We will continue to operate with a false belief about ourselves, someone else, or the world. We may feel fearful, agitated, or continually resentful. We may feel unsettled, less confident, anxious, or depressed. All of these can be symptoms of an unhealed samskara. Before we can let go, we must first bring the pattern, or samskara, to light, which involves self-awareness and a brave look inside ourselves. Breath, yoga, and tuning in all help to illuminate the samskara. Once there, we might be able to determine what is no longer serving us along our path. And then we can choose to take a different action; we can decide to start carving a new imprint.

DAY 156

Common samskaras can come from anywhere and anyone. When I was in college, I applied to be in a creative writing class. We had to submit an essay in order to be approved or rejected. My essay was rejected. The instructor also wrote a note on my essay saying I was "too verbose." I resolved never to try creative writing again. Since I had been told my writing and my voice were too wordy and shared too much, I stuck to facts. I dove into research papers and put myself into a box of unbiased information that was free from my own opinion, experience, or emotion.

I let a complete stranger tell me who I was. I took his comments on my essay as truth, not only about my writing but about myself. I hadn't thought about this interaction until I started writing my book and my blog seven years ago. I wish I would have trusted myself instead of the instructor. I wish I hadn't taken his comment personally and hadn't given up. Because my truth is this: When I write, I am more myself than when I am doing anything else in the world. When I write *verbosely* and add words, add emotions, and add my voice, I am in such a blissful state I can't imagine existing without it. I abandoned my true Self for so long.

Remember what lights you up. Remember what sets you free. Parents, teachers, siblings, and friends all may have inadvertently told you something about yourself you believed to be true. But is it true? What if you illuminate the scar? What if you stop reinforcing the belief that you are not enough, that you are too much, or that you can't?

DAY 157

We have been preparing for this process of rewriting our stories since the beginning of this book. To look at ourselves and our beliefs takes introspection, openness, and self-compassion. We need to develop trust in ourselves and trust in our body. This is why we began with practices to befriend the body—breath and movement that helped us realize our body is an ally and a teacher. We opened ourselves up to receiving intuition and listening to our heart. We observed the present moment and understood the wisdom that exists in the now. You are ready.

Even when uncomfortable emotions arrive, you know you will not break or die from feeling them. You can allow for your experience because you not only trust yourself, but you are now aware of how the mind spins and how the body responds. You are able to discern between ego narrative and truth from your higher Self. Remember, always go back to sensation. Observe without judgment. Watch without analyzing or figuring anything out. You don't have to make a list of stories you would like to rewrite. Yoga will bring everything to you and slowly show you opportunities the more you practice, the more your stay, and the more you turn inward. The practice will work on you, not the other way around.

DAY 158

Another definition of *samskara* is "rite of passage," and it means our scars are the threshold to our transformation. Samskaras are the original wound but also the antidote. By illuminating the scar, by bringing awareness to how the belief was formed, we create a new future. What was true in the past may not be true now. What we believed to be true after an experience may have never been true at all.

If you have been living with a belief about yourself and you dislike the story, consider that the belief might be your rite of passage—the story might be a threshold to creating a new belief and a new experience. Your circumstance and your past do not define you. Your tender places are teachers, and your pain is a sign of a new beginning. To heal a samskara, we can step outside of blame and victimhood and empower ourselves to walk forward with a new belief. We can recognize where we were and also where we want to go. Being treated in a way that made us feel shame in the past does not mean we need to carry that shame or guilty response with us into current situations. As children, we had no tools or wisdom in order to respond to abuse. We had no defense against adults or attacking words and actions. But today, with self-awareness, self-love, and a compassionate yoga practice that tends to our body as a small child in need of our attention, we can begin the process of uncovering abusive experiences and not allowing them to define us. Our wound is our way out.

DAY 159

What stories has your practice unearthed so far? Now that they have poked at the surface, have your beliefs created more questions? Are you noticing your stories more in your day-to-day?

Samskaras are mental imprints that dictate our beliefs and behaviors. Stories are our scars. As we move along our transformational path, uncovering and possibly rewriting our stories is a way to take responsibility for our life rather than let another person or event define us. We are not victim to what someone else says, does, or believes. We can accept hurtful, tragic, or traumatic experiences without allowing them to carry over into our current reality. This is true healing, and depending on the nature of the wound, it may require many different tools. This is not a "get over it" or "pull yourself up by your bootstraps" mentality. Yoga and the concept of samskara do not mean ignoring our experience. It's quite the opposite. Healing takes much effort and, particularly, attention to the pain something caused. Actions do affect us. And part of healing is being able to feel an experience fully so it can be processed and released. Whether over a period of time or in an instant, when we fully allow for our experience, we are able to stand in our own truth and not lose ourselves permanently because of someone else.

As I said yesterday, samskara is a rite of passage, a new path toward awakening. When we remove the layers of our conditioning and illuminate the experience, our samskaras become powerful symbols on our path to overcoming. Instead of letting someone else or some circumstance define us, we get to change the story. And we will move forward—free.

DAY 160

Stories that hold us back or play out in our lives in a detrimental way usually stem from negative self-talk or criticism from others. Someone makes a statement about who we are, and we take this belief and run with it. We hold on to a person's opinion or rude comment and allow it to be true for our entire lives.

Consider what your parents, caregivers, teachers, or bosses have told you. How have you allowed their comments to become true? If you have always believed you are "bad with money," for example, can you think of examples that prove this belief to be false? Maybe you've never dealt with finances because someone somewhere made you believe you shouldn't bother. Maybe you are actually great with money, but you've never even tried. By believing the story and acting according to it, the story is now true.

While we all have strengths and weaknesses, it's usually a stretch to think anyone is smarter, stronger, more capable, or better than anyone else. If you are walking around with a belief about your character or your capacity as a human, I bet this story is untrue—or at least deserves to be examined. *You* as a person are not flawed; you may have simply never practiced. You were told you're too loud, so you keep quiet. You were told you're too sensitive, so you dismiss your emotions. You never learned to dance because someone said you were uncoordinated.

Once we identify a story, we can practice allowing a new behavior or belief into our thoughts. It's time to form a new groove. Rake a new line in the sand.

DAY 161

Have you ever *not* gotten something you really wanted? Have you wondered why you were so unfortunate and undeserving, but then, in hindsight, you realized the thing you really wanted wasn't meant for you at all? Even though it didn't turn out how you intended, something much better and more appropriate came in—a different relationship, a different job, or a different opportunity. Looking back, you were relieved you didn't get your way. As humans, we never give ourselves enough credit. We are conditioned into believing that we are not as good as others, not as deserving, not as capable, and not as loved. We compare, and most of the time, we feel like we fall short.

So, how can we possibly know what's best for us or what's best for the greater good of humanity? We can force ourselves into jobs, relationships, cities, homes, families, and more because we are smart, resourceful, and determined. When we do get what we want, we call it fate, and when we don't get what we want, we call it failure.

What if the story you would write for yourself is far less than what you deserve? What if our tendency is to sell ourselves short? Here's the other side: Even as we have been trained to always think we could be doing more and better, our soul already knows we are perfect. Our soul already trusts there is a plan. Our soul spends a lot of time steering us in directions we don't want to go. But all directions are good; everything is leading us to what is best. Everything is leading us to our perfect, unimaginable, more-than-we-could-dream-for-ourselves *story*.

DAY 162

How do we let go of beliefs, expectations, and outcomes? How do we get out of our own way and live a life that reflects our amazing possibility rather than our small story? First, we stop worrying about the details. If we want love, for example, the possibilities of what that looks like are endless. Love can come from many people, not just the person you have in mind. The same goes for a career goal. If fulfillment or freedom is the ultimate goal, unlimited options exist. It's the details that trip us up, and what we see as an unintended path could be leading us right to where we want to be.

You have practiced enacting the observer, which is also a powerful practice in life toward any goal. Instead of forcing something into being by controlling and manipulating with no acknowledgment of how your actions affect others, be open and curious. Instead of repeating the same story—the same pattern—stop, watch, and wait. Staying curious allows us to see more clearly what might be best for us and when something we are forcing isn't really meant to be.

Lastly, remind yourself how deserving you are. Trust that the Universe has your best interests in mind as well as the best interests for all. Whatever you believe in—God, a higher power, or universal consciousness—trust that the greater good includes *you*. You are part of the plan. What you desire is waiting for you. It is overflowing, beautiful, and on its way.

DAY 163

Your entire body is energy. Physically, your body is made up of blood, veins, ligaments, muscles, and bone. Each string, each tissue, is connected and integral to the bigger system. The body is also made up of energy channels, which yoga calls *nadis*. Nadis need to be open and flowing in order to feel good and to reach our full potential. Like physical arteries that get blocked as a result of diet and lifestyle, nadis get blocked as a result of stress, lack of exercise, and when we can't handle an emotion or experience. When we are too uncomfortable or feeling too much, nadis close. We walk around the world with hidden secrets and unhealed wounds. We fail to understand the power of opening these nadis to feel better but also to acknowledge a part of ourselves that has been forgotten. Every desire, every aspect of your reality, every deep longing and heartfelt wish is a nadi waiting to be opened. For whatever reason, you shut down your experience based on someone else, a protection, a false belief, a sense of unworthiness, or fear. When nadis are purified through yoga, breath, and honest self-observation, we become more skilled at accepting difficult emotions and therefore acknowledging ourselves. Acknowledging the places where you feel sad or stuck is the first step in opening what has been holding you back so it is no longer blocked in energetic potential.

DAY 164

When I learned about nadis and samskara, my first reaction was: *I am so full of wounds, knots, and blocked energy.* My second thought was: *How do I clear it all out?*

My readiness doesn't always serve me, but here's the great news: yoga postures and mindful breathing cleanse and purify nadis without us even realizing it. Already in your practice, you're keeping nadis open and allowing your body's energy channels to flow. Your physical practice is bringing energetic benefits, keeping you healthy.

Every experience can become blocked energy if not processed and released, which creates a *granthi*, or a knot of blocked energy. In Sanskrit, *granthi* means "knot" and "doubt." These words go hand in hand. During a particularly painful experience, granthis form and are difficult to untie. We doubt our ability to feel emotions, so we close off the flow of energy. Undigested experience gets stuck in the body because we don't trust the body to heal. Every time you do yoga and every time you observe your breath, you are opening channels and undoing knots.

Healing samskara, the imprints that dictate our behavior, takes some deeper introspection. We need to be aware of the samskara in the first place, and most likely, the belief and behavior have slipped into our subconscious. It sounds so simple, but with more self-observation, you will become more self-aware. It's happening already. Just by observing the body, you've gained more trust in yourself. You have gained insight. Even off your yoga mat, you are more observant and aware in life. Knots are loosening, channels are flowing, and stories are being rewritten.

DAY 165

Today's practice uncovers a common samskara and combines meditation and journaling. Start by thinking of a story that has been coming up for you. Meditate on this story. Replay the scene in your mind. Welcome in all emotions and sensations; try to feel the experience with your entire body.

Write the story in your journal, and let your writing flow from deep inside. Don't get hung up on form or grammar; writing taps into your subconscious when you let go of what it should look like. Write a list of words, emotions, sensations, or full sentences.

Next, read the story and look for a pattern. What qualities are present in your scene? How did you feel while replaying the event? Are you scared, lonely, excited …?

Now, rewrite the story using an *opposite* quality. Begin the story with the new quality and write from there. For example, if powerlessness is a pattern in your story, write, "I am power*ful*…" and let your pen flow. What actions and behaviors are different? What sensations arrive as you rewrite the story from this new quality?

Notice I am using the word *quality* instead of *belief*. When we welcome new qualities into our experiences, we are less rigid and less judgmental. We take our beliefs to be true and unchanging, while qualities shift and change all the time. Welcome a new quality into your experience and see what happens. Welcome in love, kindness, strength, or assertiveness. Notice how the new quality affects your view of yourself or the experience. With the new quality present, how does the story change?

DAY 166

Part of rewriting and transcending our story is to stop some unhelpful behaviors and beliefs when it comes to our emotions. It is very common to want to avoid emotions altogether, especially when we label them as bad or wrong. If an emotion is present, it is meaningful. There is nothing wrong with you for having emotions, and a loving, discerning view can help to process the emotion instead of judging it and further adding to your suffering by layering on more unhelpful beliefs.

Here's a common scenario: We get mad at someone. We don't like feeling angry, so we take action to fix the emotion. We might involve the other person and tell them why we are mad. If the communication is healthy and productive, we feel better, but depending on how the interaction goes, we might feel worse. Another way to deal with the anger might be to take an inside approach. We could get curious about what caused the anger and where it's coming from. We could move, do yoga, or go for a walk to open some channels and get energy flowing. We could sit quietly and journal. Emotions not dealt with build up over time, so any one scenario might not be the sole cause for today's anger. It deserves looking at and noticing if the emotion passes with some deep breaths or mindful movement or if any new insight arrives. While it may be tempting to retaliate when someone makes us mad, this usually doesn't make us feel better in the long run, and it definitely doesn't heal the pain. It's empowering to know our choices when dealing with anger and to make the best choice for ourselves in that moment.

DAY 167

It's easy to say all emotions are equal, and in reality, they are, but obviously we like some better than others. Emotions such as loneliness, frustration, sadness, and many others arrive at unpredicted times, and we resist their presence. Something a person says or something you do or see triggers an old wound, and all of a sudden, even though you were fine a second ago, you now feel uncomfortable or disturbed. The issue is not the emotion itself but the identification with the emotion as something bad. Eckhart Tolle refers to "the knowing" as breaking free from our unconscious associations with pain. As he writes, "The knowing prevents the old emotion from rising up into your head and taking over not only the internal dialogue, but also your actions as well as interactions with other people."[40] The knowing part of us sees the emotion, acknowledges the pain it's causing, and faces the emotion head-on. We don't blame others, berate ourselves, or react maliciously. We understand the emotion is not who we are, so we practice acceptance. We stop trying to control the emotion, and we allow for it instead. Emotions stay inside our body until they are felt. If we agitate the emotion by fretting unnecessarily over it, shoving it down, or feeding it more story, the emotion is never able to pass. Once we observe an emotion for what it is—a physical sensation in the body and a reaction to experience—the emotion *will* move and release. When we free ourselves from the stories of our uncomfortable emotions, it gets a lot easier to allow and release the emotions as they arrive.

....

40. Tolle, *A New Earth*, 183.

DAY 168

I have several yoga clients who began a yoga practice while recovering from or going through cancer. Physical illness is an excellent teacher, especially a disease like cancer, which can have little explanation or direct cause. No one truly knows how to prevent it, yet patients often feel responsible for their illness. The belief is that the body has failed them, which leads to mistrust and resentment. Certainly, with my addiction to alcohol, I felt responsibility and shame. Our addiction makes us act in regrettable ways, and we think the disease is a result of being a bad person. The beliefs we hold about ourselves when facing physical illness or injury are important to uncover. I remind my clients with cancer that it is helpful to address any feelings of shame, powerlessness, or fear that arrive during their diagnosis or recovery. It can be easy to blame or chastise the body as weak or inadequate when facing certain physical illnesses. The body becomes ill due to physical, environmental, and many other factors, and how we treat ourselves during recovery affects our ability to heal. Instead of pushing fears and doubts away, lean into these feelings. Meet the cancer or illness head-on with radical acceptance and eventually love. A body in recovery deserves tenderness and care, not criticism. Once my clients start to treat themselves with more kindness instead of worrying about what they could have done differently, they are better able to make it through their illness and any outcomes with acceptance, grace, and true healing. Accepting any physical ailment can be the first step to accepting our whole Self. We are not separate from the body, even when the body is sick.

DAY 169

Imagine if your body never digested food or engaged in processes of elimination. Imagine all that would be stuck and built up. Our body is able to release emotions the same way it digests food; we take what we need for nourishment, and we eliminate the rest. In twelve-step recovery models, people engage in a personal inventory, an empowering step to "change ourselves to meet conditions," rather than be at the whim of others without any responsibility. [41]

Many people resist this step because they fear facing a regret or painful moment from their past. Some experiences we simply wish never would have happened, so what's the point in going back?

Actually, there is much to be gained from assessing our experience. Our ability to look within holds all our power and unlocks our transformation. By taking stock of ourselves, we can see where misperception, anger, victimhood, or fear have played a role in our current experience. Writing down my list of fears and resentments unburdened me of so much I had been carrying. The act of making a list was like being heard and seen for the first time. My ego slowly shifted into the background as I allowed myself to pour out onto the page. Things I had been holding on to out of guilt or a refusal to admit my anger didn't seem so scary once I read them. They seemed human; they seemed real. Admitting my list was uncomfortable, but becoming aware of how I could change moving forward was worth it.

. . . .

41. *Twelve Steps and Twelve Traditions*, 47.

DAY 170

Rewriting our stories is challenging, painful work. It takes a lot of courage and a lot of coming back to yourself when you might want to run the other way. If you're experiencing any resistance to your yoga practice or your spiritual practice, know that this is normal when you start to dive into some deep and transformative stuff.

I want you to take a moment to celebrate all the times you've shown up on your yoga mat, even if it's the last place you've wanted to be. Celebrate the days your practice has been profound and the days your practice has been so-so. Welcome it all in. Acknowledge your whole experience as the culmination—the entire shift from when you first began.

Where are you stronger? Where are you more flexible? What has changed off your mat, including relationships, beliefs, or self-talk? Where can you see light and hope that didn't exist before?

Most of the time we can't see how far we've come. We focus on where we are still stuck. We expect that we should be further along. Despite all our effort and commitment, we still focus on what isn't working or how we are not meeting our own expectations. The truth is that any small movement forward is a giant leap in the world of transformation. Any small change in routine, like adding yoga and meditation to your day, is monumental. And maybe you're seeing your yoga practice seep into other areas of your life as well. If you're here and practicing, I am giving you a big, warm hug. Please remember how amazing you are.

DAY 171

Our bodies and our psyches are in a constant state of growth and change. We could be moving through a monumental life event, such as a loved one's death, or we could be trying to recover from an embarrassing moment at work. Regardless, we have an experience, we process it, and we move on. Processing can look like many different things, require various tools, and take any length of time. Different people can be involved in the same exact experience, like a car accident, and recover from the event in very different ways. There is no right or good way. Everyone is different, so there is no need to compare your journey to anyone else's.

As we've learned from samskara, a current experience can jostle up dust from our past. When I discovered my husband's affair, I felt unbearable sadness. I could also call it grief, fear of the unknown, or slamming into reality. *Do you know those moments?* The world stops, and you are so close to presence, you wonder how the rest of the world is functioning as if everything is normal. During my moment of painful clarity, I was simultaneously brought back to a friend's death that happened several years before. Her death awakened these same emotions: the unknown, the preciousness of life, and my powerlessness. It was as if these two experiences were intertwined. Despite happening many years apart, these separate events pressed on the same wound. They illuminated the samskara. They brought me right here—to touch what is real—to this moment, this life, and this body. All the love and all the pain flew to the surface. Could I stay and honor my experience?

DAY 172

Even once we commit and know our path forward, things will arrive that threaten to pull us under or make us want to quit. For whatever reason, my divorce and my addiction both surfaced in the same year. Sometimes, we listen to the subtle whispers that tell us something is getting out of control, and other times, everything comes crashing to a head all at once. Navigating both experiences has felt a lot like drowning, treading water, floating for a bit on a smooth surface, sinking back down, and bobbing up for air.

Divorce doesn't end when the final papers are signed. Ending a committed relationship means learning an entirely new life without someone you thought would be there. I had waves of confidence followed by doubts when bills were due or I had to spend a holiday alone. I wondered if I had made the right decision or if it would have been easier to stay. My recovery began as a never-ending dark night of willpower, fighting each day to stay sober. Slowly, sobriety became more natural, and I experienced the magic of life without numbing. Free from substance, I could be present and breathe. I learned to face emotions and discovered that I wouldn't die from feeling pain.

Neither my divorce nor my recovery have been smooth sailing. But rough waters along the way doesn't mean my choices were wrong. I've learned to live one day at a time, to keep at it, and eventually, the days have built into an entire new existence. Trust your choice. Honor your commitment, and know that the best, most meaningful decisions aren't always the smoothest—at least not until you get the hang of it.

DAY 173

A myth around any overcoming is that we are done learning at the first sign of success. Ending a bad habit or going through a difficult life change has a lot of challenges at first. The beginning of the journey is when we get out of our comfort zone and step into the unfamiliar. This first step is huge—many people don't take it. After the first step, we keep going, and often, the new way of life feels worse before it feels better. So, what in us makes us continue? Our resilience. Our inner knowing. It is our gut that reminds us this is right. We are on the path.

All of life is a practice, and anything worthwhile requires discipline and a continued returning. At first, we glimpse freedom and possibility and then are quickly dragged back to an old way of being. It takes time and continued practice to undo years of acting a different way. All we know is the old life and the old behaviors; how unreasonable to think a lifetime of beliefs can be undone and dismantled in a short amount of time. The more times we return to ourselves and our practice, the more our successes will become more noticeable and last much longer. We might not be dragged as quickly back to the old way. There are lessons in the overcoming and on the path of imperfection. Soon, your new practice will become comfortable and familiar, and you will walk the new line with ease.

DAY 174
Balance

*Stand on one leg. Observe your body adjust to hold the balance.
Your supporting foot presses down and wobbles side to side. Your
core tightens into action and pulls you back each time you waver.
Your arms find a helpful extension.*

Standing balance postures teach us so much about resilience and
what can be learned when we fall. Just like the body constantly moves
and adjusts, tilting and wobbling to stay upright, so, too, does our practice in life. Every time we fall out, every time we lose our balance, we
learn something precious about our journey. When we practice balance,
muscles develop memory, strength, and skill. Just like uncovering and
rewriting stories, balance takes some falling out and coming back. The
body learns from every recovery. If you have resigned to the inaccurate
belief of *I am terrible at balance*, consider how you're using and distrib-
uting your energy. Balance requires equal parts ease and effort. Just like
other life lessons, we cannot will our body to remain in the pose; the
body learns through mistakes and sensation. We become familiar with
balance when we become familiar with imbalance. As we tip and try,
we learn which muscles are necessary for balance and which can stay at
ease. Reaching through the crown of the head, for example, and finding
more length supports your standing foot. Clenching your jaw and yelling at yourself does not support your effort. Breathing helps the body
relax. Lowering the shoulders shifts the heart into alignment. Balance
is discovering where your energy is best distributed and getting familiar
with sensations of ease and effort—just like rewriting stories.

DAY 175

Doubt sets in. It's usually when we have a setback or a supposed failure—usually when we are tired or worn down. That's when the small voice sees an opportunity to make us quit. It's the voice that tells us we can't, we shouldn't, or *"What were we thinking?!"* When we are at our most vulnerable, we can give in to the voice.

Whether I'm parenting, teaching yoga, or working toward any goal, the critical voice is there. I've realized this voice will never leave my thought process, but there are ways I can manage and quiet the voice when it arrives. We all have that voice. We all experience self-doubt. We all fear failure and crave an easier solution to our problems. Most everything worthwhile requires staying, consistency, and not giving up or giving in—especially not giving in to the voice that tells you to quit, that you're not worthy, or whatever else floats into your head during times of personal growth and progress.

The trick with this inner critic is to acknowledge that it's there and know that the voice is not accurate or wise. Your critical voice may show up on your yoga mat or in your life. Notice when it shows up. Observe the critical voice and look for patterns. Chronic negative self-talk points to our beliefs, and knowing those beliefs is the first step to flipping them.

DAY 176

I believe that if there is something you are trying to achieve or something you are trying to stick to, you absolutely can; there is no reason you can't do something you put your heart into. Most of the time, when people don't achieve something, it's because they give up. They decide they don't really want it anymore, or they decide it's too much effort and too much pain. There are a million excuses. We trick ourselves into believing the particular path is not for us when, in reality, we may just be giving up.

The beat of your heart tells you to keep going. Listen to that. Tell the doubting voice you have everything you need. Tell yourself you are worthy, deserving, and capable. Take heart in these words from Buddhist teacher Pema Chödrön: "To stay with that shakiness— to stay with a broken heart, with a rumbling stomach, with the feeling of hopelessness and wanting to get revenge—that is the path of true awakening."[42] We spend too much time feeding and fearing our own self-doubt. Truthfully, not much can be avoided if we just keep at it.

Staying teaches us lessons along the way. Staying tells the Universe we are serious. Staying builds our character and our resolve. Staying strengthens our heart and our resilience instead of strengthening the voice that says we can't. You can. I can. We all can. I believe that nothing is out of reach for you unless you stop reaching.

....
42. Chödrön, *When Things Fall Apart*, 11.

DAY 177

Our life is cloaked in stories based on experience. When something validates our story, it makes the groove that much deeper and the story that much more believable. Our stories create habits that turn into addictions and obsessions. Our stories prevent us from taking risks. They keep us comfortable and tethered to the material world and all its illusions. Our stories keep us small because as long as our ego tells us we are unworthy, lacking, and not enough, it holds all the power. What stories have you been telling yourself?

One of my stories when I was little was: *If I can keep adults happy, nothing bad will happen.* So, I smiled and obliged and took on the insane burden of making others happy, even at the expense of myself. Smiling faces became my security blanket, and anything else induced fear and guilt. Of course *all stories are illusions*, which means we can let our stories go. If you could let go of one story, what would it be?

Free yourself from one story. Say it out loud, write it down, and remind yourself throughout the day. It *will* come up, and you'll realize how often you revert to the story and how much it doesn't serve you. I give you permission; you are free to let it go.

DAY 178

Look around your home, your workplace, or your environment. The people, places, items, and emotions that surround you have all been welcomed in by you. Maybe there are pieces of your life that feel like obligations or necessities rather than choices. To acknowledge your life as your choice is not meant to pile on guilt or regret. To acknowledge your life as your choice actually brings incredible power and ownership. Owning your life and your situation means you can change it.

Obligations are usually illusions based on fear. Necessities are usually the result of narrow-minded thinking and small beliefs, which are also rooted in fear. Our fear of doing something different or belief that there isn't a different way prevents us from seeing alternative and greater possibilities. Sometimes, we create a life that we are told will fulfill us only to find out we want something else or something different. We are sold many images of happiness and success, but the reality is that we still need to choose for ourselves. Our happiness is dependent on our unique gifts and our personal truth. Most of the time, we are not victims like we think. Our excuses, which keep us stuck, are not so valid. Consider stories you tell yourself that keep you from making a change. Is there a way to open a little around your story and see your situation from a wider view? Your life is your choice. You can make a small change and take one step in order to get closer to the life you want. As you move along, more will be revealed, and you will discover new possibilities and options along the way. Your confidence will grow as you realize how limited your thinking was.

DAY 179

At the beginning of any new adventure, be it a relationship, a career, a physical or mental health journey, relocating, or pursuing a passion, it's impossible to see all the benefits and growth that awaits. We might set a goal to stop eating sugar with the expectation that we will lose weight or feel better, but we have no idea that this small change will ripple into other more beautiful things such as our self-confidence, our relationships, or our mindset. One of the hardest parts about changing a habit is letting go of the beliefs we attach to it. Often, you can't imagine feeling happy or content with a new habit or routine. You can't imagine how you would change the pattern or what would replace it.

When I quit drinking, I could not see past the actual alcohol. I couldn't imagine parties, weddings, dinners, events, weekends, or holidays without it. How would any of those be fun? Over time, I learned all of life is fun sober; I was only living in the illusion that alcohol had anything to do with it. This is an example of a false belief and an excuse based on fear. In addition to learning that life could be fun without drinking, I also had no idea of the amazing people and opportunities that would fill my life once I got sober. I have friends I never would have had. I have strength I never knew existed. Things have come into my life that I never expected. My choice to stop drinking not only fixed an immediate problem but brought so many new and exhilarating possibilities. The small change in belief you are working on now will snowball into so much more.

DAY 180

It's impossible to grasp the orchestration and meaning behind every single relationship, encounter, mundane decision, and big life experience. I believe people and situations are all brought into our life for a reason. And the cool thing is that just as the Universe is always conspiring for your benefit, it also conspires for everyone else's benefit, too, which means we are all in this together, helping each other in our lessons, in our inspiration, in our personal growth, and along our paths.

A difficult conversation with someone, an argument, or a breakup are all opportunities to learn something about ourselves, and given that another person is involved, we are probably helping them do the same. I have regrets. There are experiences from my past I wish weren't there, and there are experiences where I wish I had known better. But the truth is: *How could I have known better when I hadn't yet been through it?* Maybe that very person, situation, or event was there to teach me what I needed to learn so that I wouldn't repeat the same mistake or go down a certain path at all. If we trust that the events in our life, even the ones we don't like or aren't proud of, were necessary for our growth, then we can let go of our attachment to those events in order to move forward. We don't have to be tied to our past. We can remain aware of it and carry the lessons but not the guilt or the pain.

The only reason you are the person you are today is because of every life experience up to this point. There are no perfect paths. The "imperfect" paths bring us exactly what we need when we make the choice to become self-aware and to grow.

DAY 181

A culmination means something is attained, something is lost, and something awaits. Culmination brings everything to a peak that's maybe in the form of a goal being reached or a life stage completing. These moments of extreme pointedness, when we can clearly see the end of something that was and the start of something new, unsettle us. Our awareness of life and death—of endings and beginnings—is not necessarily comfortable.

An example might be shedding physical weight from the body. A person who experiences significant weight loss often feels a sense of loss for their former Self. Despite wanting to lose weight, the body that identified them for so long is no longer here. Hence, grief shows up along with joy, pride, and accomplishment. Emotional shedding is similar. Letting go of unhealthy beliefs and habits is like death. We can fight for something for so long, whether it's recovering from an illness, battling an addiction, or working toward a life goal, that our very identity becomes tied to the process.

Pretty soon, we are defined by the illness, by the recovery, or by the project. Then, when we do reach our goal, it feels oddly unfamiliar. We are used to working *toward* the outcome, not being there, at the end, as the receiver. Cancer patients describe a new identity once they recover. Addicts experience a letting go of lifestyle and their sense of Self. New parents navigate the loss of their former Self before children. Do we allow ourselves to feel and grieve the loss, whatever it is? Can we admit that joy, sadness, fear, and excitement all exist at the peak, the culmination?

DAY 182

The stories we write for ourselves are out of protection. They served us in the past. The question we must ask is: *What serves us now?* Past experience has a way of remaining in our soul and our psyche, so we keep our walls up long after the experience has passed. We don't want to feel that way ever again. How do we not let our past define us forever?

Enter bravery. Bravery is when we move forward into something that has caused us pain in the past and when we do it knowing full well that we could get hurt. Bravery is when we continue to operate with an open heart despite past cracks and bruises. There are so many ways in life we can practice the vulnerability it takes to be brave. We implement boundaries with friends and loved ones. We move forward into new relationships after heartbreak. We put our dream on the line, even when the future is unknown and we know we might fail.

Our bravery inspires others to be brave, and we heal each other along the way. To be in this life is to be affected by our past. Our past can be traumatic or not; regardless, our past shapes us. Our past has the power to shut us down from love, from ourselves, and from life—forever. The only way to reshape the past is to enter situations that may trigger us and notice how we react. It might be painful. It might burn and ache. But if we can move through the trigger, if we can ride the wave of emotion without jumping off, we can overcome the past and create a new future.

DAY 183

In exploring our samskaras, we have been looking at personal stories that may be holding us back. These are stories that were necessary at some point, but today, they can be rewritten in order to honor our true Self now, not the version from the past. We can take our practice further into the world by noticing how our stories and beliefs have been shaped not only by our individual experience but also by the overall culture in which we live.

As a woman, I carry the collective scars of society's beliefs and representations of all women. Marginalized groups carry oppressive beliefs that may not be theirs—beliefs that are the result of an entire society's actions. Consider how your stories might be personal and also shared. Like all samskaras, we do not need to accept the beliefs imposed by society as truth.

Healing starts with you, but your healing also has the power to heal the stories of society, of institutions, and of a culture. Without realizing it, we perform certain actions based on society's conditioning, not necessarily out of personal choice.

What would it look like to illuminate a collective scar so we can finally be free of it? Would it look like empathy for someone else's experience? Would it look like understanding? Would it look like change?

We not only owe it to ourselves; we owe it to the world to bring our beliefs and actions into awareness and questioning, even under a bright spotlight and even when it is painful or possibly offensive. Like all our practices, rewriting stories is about you—and also greater humanity.

PRACTICE 7
Ungrasping (Aparigraha)

Sanskrit words have multiple meanings, and sometimes, the meaning cannot even be sufficiently translated into an English word. *Aparigraha*, for example, translates to "nonattachment," "nonpossessiveness," and my favorite—"ungrasping." We really don't have common words in English that mean the same as aparigraha because our culture does not practice the concept. Our cultural norm is to amass great wealth, status, and possessions in order to feel fulfilled. The closest we have to an English translation of *aparigraha*, which encompasses all its meanings, is "to let go." To practice aparigraha does not mean we stop having expectations, goals, dreams, or desires. It means we learn how to detach from a particular image or outcome in order to experience fully what is and to welcome in boundless possibility.

DAY 184

What does it mean to ungrasp? To loosen our grip, to stop hanging on so tightly? I picture the ropes course I did in high school where I teetered on a single rope strung high between two trees. There were ropes of different lengths hanging above me to help me get across. But in order to reach the next rope, to progress along the tightrope and make it to the other side, I had to briefly let go of the rope behind me. There was simply too much distance for my arms to grab both ropes at the same time. As much as I tried, I could not get to the next rope on the line without first letting go of the one behind me.

For a moment, I was suspended. For a moment, I had no rope to hold on to for balance. For a moment, I had to trust. This is the practice of aparigraha. It is to feel fulfilled and trusting—even when we have nothing solid to attach to. Most of our grasping comes from a desire for permanence. We feel something uplifting, like new love or swelling pride from an accomplishment, and we want the feeling to last forever. So, we cling to the fear that we will lose the feeling, and we try to manufacture it over and over again. We refuse to let go or loosen our grip, even when letting go of the past is what we need to progress forward.

DAY 185

I have always wanted a map to fall into my lap and tell me what to do, especially when I am in turmoil. The Eight Limbs of Yoga actually offer a pretty detailed design for living a complete and fulfilled life. Each limb is a guide and a practice on the road to enlightenment. The first limb contains the five yamas, yoga's five moral restraints that shift our thoughts. Aparigraha is one of the five yamas, an ethical practice that helps us experience more joy and less turmoil. The five yamas are nonviolence, truth, nonstealing, nonexcess, and nonattachment (aparigraha).

We can apply any of the five yamas to any life situation and gain clarity. If we are experiencing pain or suffering, we may be dishonoring one of the suggested restraints. For example, when it comes to aparigraha, are we attached to a certain outcome that is preventing us from seeing other possibilities? Are we stuck in the illusion that things should stay the same? Are we unwilling to let go of something that has run its course? Are we clinging to security and fearful of the unknown?

Let us set our minds and our hearts on the practice of aparigraha. Practicing nonattachment liberates us from outside circumstance and material weight. Aparigraha helps you enjoy life while knowing that when something leaves you (or you leave it), there is always something else ready and waiting.

DAY 186

Do you want to progress across the tightrope, or do you want to keep holding on? Do you want to be tied to an expectation and continually live in fear that something won't happen? Do you want to remain stuck in unforgiveness, surrounded by possessions, and attached to an old belief about yourself? Do you want to keep hoarding money and things that constantly require more and more to sustain? I love this quote by Deborah Adele: "Anything we cling to creates a maintenance problem for us."[43]

A relationship can bring us joy and fulfillment. A delicious meal can bring us flavor and contentment. Career success can bring us confidence and validation. But all people and circumstances in life are temporary and ever changing. Thus, we need more stuff, more success, or more praise in order to maintain what something outside ourselves brings us. Nonattachment teaches us that the emotions we crave actually come from within. Our self-worth, self-acceptance, and self-confidence do not depend on outside validation. They exist regardless of our situation, which means we can become more skilled at letting go when the next rope is waiting for us. Even if there is a moment of temporary doubt and suspension into the unknown, letting go with grace and faith will always bring us to the next level of support and the next exhilarating opportunity.

....
43. Adele, *The Yamas & Niyamas*, 95.

DAY 187

A lot of our personal and spiritual growth gets stunted when we cling to bad memories or regrets from the past or when we worry about plans or expectations in the future, when we place expectations on others, or when we demand specific outcomes. The practice of presence frees us from the past and the future, so we can experience joy and fulfillment in the current moment. In a sense, the past and the future only exist in your mind; they're inside whatever story you are making up about something that is not currently happening. The present moment is the only thing that is real. Touch it. Feel it. Try not to judge it. What is your experience right now, and can you be with it?

As we continue to practice aparigraha (nonattachment and ungrasping), I invite you to notice how often you allow the present moment to be your reality. Most of us live entirely in the past or in the future; we tend to lean into regret or unforgiveness, or we spend our time obsessing about something that has yet to occur. If you live mostly in the future, you may also spend time hoping that someone will change, hoping that you will change, or daydreaming about how your life would be different "if only" or "when." You live in the future instead of appreciating the now. Don't wait to start living. Let go of the past and recognize your accomplishments today. Let go of the future and begin your journey right now, even if you don't feel ready. The heaviness of what we cling to keeps us stuck when we are actually free—free to enjoy ourselves *right now*.

DAY 188

The day I quit drinking was not my last day. Of course I wanted it to be, but that wasn't my path. After each relapse, I got stuck in the regret and shame of not staying completely sober from the start. This shame and regret could have prevented me from getting up and trying again. In order to move on, I had to let go of what was behind me and keep looking forward. Clinging to any painful past experience can severely limit our possibilities moving forward. Beliefs like *"I'm better off alone so I don't get hurt,"* *"The world is dangerous; I can't trust,"* and *"I am not cut out for this profession"* will prevent us from realizing our future.

In brand-new sobriety, I often got frustrated with the present moment. I wanted to be further along. I wanted to "get it." But the only way to make progress is by walking forward one day at a time. Little by little, by accepting where we are each day, we gain confidence and wisdom. Nothing can be gained without an acknowledgment and an acceptance of the present moment. This is true in relationships, careers, parenting, and spiritual growth. Just like in yoga, we need to arrive where we are; we don't expect to know a pose fully without trying and faltering several times along the way. Then, one day, we hold a balance longer than ever before, or we find that our heels are meeting the ground in downward-facing dog. All our efforts and our practice pay off when we realize that by accepting ourselves each day, we have made life-changing progress over time.

DAY 189

How can we care about a person, relationship, outcome, family situation, health issue, career goal, or shiny new car and still not be *attached*? The practice of aparigraha does not mean we stop caring about people or outcomes. The practice of aparigraha actually allows us to care more deeply and fully for what is happening now instead of what we want something to be. To practice aparigraha is to live completely in the moment and to let that moment fulfill us instead of the expectation of something "else."

How often have you dragged a heavy load of worry with you into a job interview, a first date, a plane trip, a doctor's appointment, or a situation with an outcome that is out of your control? How often have you tried to grab control of a situation, a person, or yourself in order to feel secure that the circumstance won't slip away or change? We falsely believe our attachments bring us peace and happiness, but in reality, they keep us caged. Rather than gain freedom by grabbing for control, we simply gain more work. There is a big difference between caring and carrying. We can care without clinging. We can acknowledge disappointment, resentment, frustration, or fear while also staying open and curious. We can be with the moment when we recognize our emotions as a reaction to attachment. We unburden ourselves when we soften around the attachment and get curious about what wants to arrive.

DAY 190

A person we trust hurts us, betrays us, or disappoints us. Our heart breaks, and we never want to feel that pain again. Our solution is to close, to not put ourselves out there, as a way to protect ourselves. Closing your heart as the result of a past hurt is a form of attachment. By not freeing ourselves from our past, we are not living a fully present or true experience. Yes, letting go might be vulnerable and raw, and you might get hurt, but to never experience pain or heartache is not the point. We are able to enjoy a relationship more fully when we let go of the fear that we will get hurt. We are able to enjoy our children or elderly parents more fully when we let go of the idea that life needs to stay this way. We are able to enjoy all experiences in their purest states when we place our mind in the experience itself and not in the illusion of control.

It is possible to appreciate the present without all our shields of protection. The things we carry—the past, the pain, the incident, the belief, the pattern—all become slowly familiar, and we learn to cling to them rather than release our grip. The familiar feels like home, even if it is restricting, even if it prevents us from another opportunity. Getting hurt does not need to keep you from giving or receiving love in the future. Screwing up does not need to stop you from trying again. This is a way of staying attached to the pain instead of being free from it. When you are ready, it is possible to let your past go.

DAY 191

The concept of ungrasping is underused in our Western society. I remember the first time I ever read the word. My fingers immediately uncurled, and my jaw lost its clench. It was like being given a grand permission; I realized I didn't have to try so hard. We fear we will lose something if we release our grip. We fear that if we get rid of our expectation, a relationship, situation, or outcome will not turn out how we want. We forget about faith—faith in the greater good, faith in ourselves, and faith in others.

Just like we need physical exercise in order to change and strengthen our bodies, our mental muscles need strengthening too. We can change behaviors, thoughts, patterns, and emotions. Our mental state and our responses and reactions will become more natural with practice. In yoga, we continue to ask questions in order to remove layers of false belief and conditioning. When we ask questions, we start to see that maybe we don't need what has held us captive after all. We might be able to try something new, change our route, or unload a box at the donation center. As we learn to let go through practice and see that the world doesn't come crashing in on us, we become more comfortable relying on something outside ourselves instead of our own control. Ungrasping gives us permission to soften, and we move through life with more ease. We don't have to try so hard to force everything into an idea we think is best. We then don't need to get so disappointed when our idea doesn't work out. Imagine the softening and the freedom of not hanging on so tightly.

DAY 192

Take out your journal and consider these prompts on letting go. As always, write freely and from your heart, without the restriction of grammar or form.

- List roles or labels you associate with yourself. Some examples are mother, teacher, victim, peacekeeper, or best friend.
- List qualities you attach to each of these roles. Some examples are nurturing, fearful, brave, kind, loyal, or smart.
- Free write as you explore these questions.
  - What does this role allow me to do and be?
  - How do I benefit?
  - Without this role, what could I no longer do?
- What would I have to do/change if I was no longer defined by this role? Some examples are speak up, say no, put myself out there, set boundaries, take care of myself, be honest, get a job, or find something to do with my time.
- Write emotions or reactions that come up with your list of changes. Do you see a pattern? What scares you, and what is preventing you from letting this go?

We all get attached to our roles because they are very comfortable. We adopt positive, healthy qualities but also negative and sometimes damaging qualities from the roles we play. It helps to look at our roles and determine if the behavior or belief attached to the role is serving us or if the belief or behavior is keeping us stuck and preventing us from stepping into a new experience.

DAY 193
Letting Go Meditation

Begin seated on your mat or in a chair. Close your eyes. With your hands resting on your knees, curl your fingers into your palms and squeeze your hands into tight fists. Continue holding the fists as you breathe long, slow, and even. Bring to mind something you know you are attached to. You can choose an everyday object, a job offer, or an emotion or story you are tired of seeing come up. Hold this attachment tightly inside your palms. Squeeze harder around the attachment, imagining how much you need it to exist. On the next exhale, slowly, lovingly, and with care, allow your fingers to open. Let the exhale be long and liquid as your hands open and you release your grip on your attachment. Sit with your hands face up on your knees and continue to breathe. Notice how you feel.

This meditation is a great practice to get a sense of what we hold on to and any fears around letting it go. It might be hard to open your fists at first. Your body might react in fear. You might feel great relief as your palms open and you no longer have to hold on to the emotion, person, or outcome. Notice. Complete this practice as often as you need and with different attachments. You should gain much insight. Once you uncurl your fists, once you release your grip, you do not have to pick the attachment up again. You can be free.

DAY 194

There is something you've been holding tightly on to, and you can now *let it go*.

You don't yet know who you will be without this thing because it has been a part of you for a long time. Trust that your body knows when it is time to let go. Trust that anything arriving during yoga, meditation, or in life is there for a reason. Don't turn away. Find out who this visitor is and what they want.

Our body and our heart speak to us. Our body might wince at a particular word or pose, and it's difficult to understand what the sensation means. As you read the words *let it go*, what comes up?

For me, letting go feels scary and unnatural. If I let go, how will everything work out? Letting go doesn't mean we feel great right away; we may still experience grief and sadness for what has been. There are times I still sense defeat, sadness, and heartache from my past. It's hard to think back on my marriage and other ended relationships. It's hard *not* to carry past regrets and fears into current relationships. This is what I carry—the weighted guilt of my past that I just can't let go. Letting go does not mean something won't creep up again—sometimes when we least expect it. An emotion will tug, and we can listen. With every acknowledgment and with every exhale, we can soften a little more. We can practice this until the pangs from our past don't hold as much weight and the load we carry becomes a little lighter and, therefore, easier to let go.

DAY 195

Letting go involves an amount of trust in something outside our-selves. If we do let go, will something else really arrive? Or will the letting go leave us empty, alone, and uncared for? If we let go, how will anything get resolved? Don't we have to keep at it? Keep tend-ing? Keep checking? Keep making sure?

The answer is no. Think about the seeds beneath the earth in winter. No one can see all that is happening underneath. In fact, the only way to tell if the seeds actually took is when the stems and flowers arrive in spring.

I love a quiet snowfall on a dark winter night. White glitter drops silently down, landing on the ground and bare tree branches, a prom-ise of protection despite the supposed lack of growth. To me, new snowfall is the promise of a clean slate and endless possibility.

Whatever you are holding, ungrasp. You will be catapulted to your true intention, and you will be given a new chance. Like the warm blanket of snow over seeds that are quietly stirring under-neath, your heart's desire is germinating. Trust that the letting go is working. Trust that the flowers will arrive. The energy is already churning, and even if you have no proof yet, the promise of a new beginning is imprinting into your reality, like footprints on the never-been-walked-on, newly fallen snow.

DAY 196

It is difficult to meet our expectations; they also keep us tied to a narrow view. Whether the expectations are our own, society's, or someone else's, we place a lot of weight on them, which can be disastrous if reality doesn't match the image in our head. It took my life falling apart for me to understand that my expectations were a cage I kept myself in. I tried for so long to keep propping things up and pasting things back together, such as my marriage, my addiction, and my inner feelings and desires. I felt if I just kept the image of meeting the expectation going, then I would feel better. No one would think I had failed.

The expectations become a never-ending chase and constant struggle. We miss out on other opportunities and possibilities because we are so focused on living up to our version. We stay too long in relationships, jobs, and unhealthy habits because we are too afraid of what life will look like if we let go.

When I woke up divorced, sober, happy, peaceful, inspired, trusting, and hopeful, I thought about how much all my expectations had weighed me down. My life looks completely different than I would have pictured, but every single wonderful, painful, life-shattering, soul-searching, heartbreaking, thrilling, loving, miraculous thing that has ever happened to me has led me here. All my expectations only served to keep me suffering more than I had to. In addition to any emotional turmoil already going on, my fear of not meeting the expectation created further inner turmoil. What would it look like for you to release expectations? Maybe just one? Which expectation is heaviest? Which one is not serving you? Set it free.

DAY 197

Only when we look back on difficult situations we have overcome, do we gain the perspective of wisdom and understanding. Nothing feels fair or reasonable in moments of despair and confusion. But if we can trust ourselves and trust that we are meant to grow, learn, and change, evolving little by little as we move through a challenging time, that faith will keep us going.

So, wherever you are right now, everything that led up to this moment was necessary. Just like everything that arrives after this moment will also be part of your individual path and your individual awakening. Yoga teaches us that all experiences are felt and processed in the body. Resisting an experience is the same as refusing to let it go. Ignoring an emotion or situation does not make it disappear. The body holds on—whether the mind addresses it or not.

Your experience is happening; you must stay in it if you want it to move. Of course we have choices. We do hold the power to change the course of our life. This can be a change in belief or behavior. If there is a pattern, a relationship, a job, or a situation that we don't like, we have the choice to shift. We only know our choices when we observe what is happening right now, not from a place of judgment, victimhood, or hopelessness but from a place of absolute power and acceptance for what is.

DAY 198

While we are certainly affected by other people's actions toward us, things done *to* us do not have to define who we are—at least not in a way that keeps us small and undeserving. Challenges can be the catalyst for great change, necessary change. They can coax us into a new perspective, a new learning experience, and a new way to help others. Likewise, we should admit how our own choices have affected our path and make changes as we see fit. We can let go of a person while also forgiving them. We can set a boundary in order to take responsibility for our part. Any adjustment in course can only be good enough for right now. A year from today, you might want to make a different choice. Treat yourself with kindness and compassion and allow for changing your mind. The promise of impermanence means everything is always changing and growing, deepening and expanding. Consider something you have been in long term—a romantic relationship, family, or career. It has changed as you have changed.

Consider parts of your past you are grateful for, even if they caused great pain at the time. Observe how you have grown from them, and with the gift of hindsight, can you acknowledge any benefits? Gratitude for all parts of your experience is a powerful practice in letting go of victimhood and embracing trust in the bigger plan. We can only control how we move through something, not the actions of others. Take with you the lessons, and let go of the tendency to internalize problems as something inherently wrong with you. The past is a teacher for this moment. It is not a punishment and not an absolute.

DAY 199

Healing can take place in an instant. Sometimes, you are just done—*enough*. You end the unhealthy, destructive behavior, and you never look back. Often, however, healing and transformation is gradual and a result of a continued practice or discipline. We start small, and we start with one step, one day at a time. Each new step, each new behavior, goes against our deeply embedded samskara, and we begin to fill in the groove.

I returned to my yoga practice after a hiatus of about six years. The practice brought me to the truth that I needed to quit drinking. Of all the answers I wanted, this was not one of them, but I knew drinking was destroying my body, numbing parts of me that longed to be heard, and keeping me stuck in a samskara. Alcohol was shockingly hard to let go of, not only physically but emotionally. I had the substance on such a pedestal and attached to so many beliefs about fun, celebration, and my own identity. We can cling to our painful pasts and healing journeys just like we can cling to the good and fulfilling things in our life. Our past and our pain is familiar and therefore comfortable.

At some point during your journey, it's okay to simply say, *"I'm done. Enough."* Consider where you are grasping and hanging on. Trust your own heart. Let your wise Self emerge to reveal the answers. Your reality is your current circumstance, but you are able to grow into something new or change your situation if you have the courage to bravely let go.

DAY 200

Any door closed, any decision made, can be opened again by us at a future time. Decisions are meant to serve the moment, and they might need to be adjusted as the circumstance changes. Part of the overwhelm we feel when making a decision is the belief that it has to be final or forever. Often, life makes decisions for us or at least nudges us in a direction we might not have considered. An illness, the loss of a job, a pandemic, or an unexpected event forces our hand. In the moment, we do the best we can with the information and the circumstance in front of us. Life continually changes. People change. Jobs change. Situations change. We change. So, our decisions must change as well.

When I got sober, I had to make many tough choices. My recovery had to come first, and everything else took a back seat for the time being. I attempted to rid myself and my life of all things that caused undo stress. I simplified. I let things go. I went to tons of therapy sessions and tons of recovery meetings. I had zero social life.

I didn't understand that my recovery would not always require so much focused attention. At the time, I needed solid routine and firm boundaries. As my strength grew and I felt more settled, I gave myself permission to revisit my boundaries. Changing a career path does not mean you can never go back. Ending a hobby does not mean you can't start again. Moving to a new city does not mean you can never come home. Some doors are meant to stay closed. Some might ask you to reconsider. Trust that you are flexible.

DAY 201

The times that have been the biggest growth moments for me have never been convenient. But then, is there a convenient time to focus on our mental health? Is there a convenient time to get divorced? Is there a convenient time to make any big change? The things that will catapult us forward are rarely convenient because if it were up to us, we'd probably just stay the same—comfortable and in our normal routine.

The things that will catapult us forward almost always appear sudden. Truthfully, they've built up over time, nudging us slowly at first, until something more eventful forces us to actually wake up and pay attention. I believe that timing is both perfect and inconvenient—always. Whatever is happening for you right now, it is time. Time to do what's necessary. Time to take care of yourself. Time to say no. Time to say yes. Time to embark on a new adventure. Time to quit. Time to allow your heart to open. Time to choose yourself.

Whatever is uncomfortable is here to teach you something. It is here to grab your attention. If it's happening, you don't need to worry about whether or not it's the right time. If it's happening, it *is* time. This is true for good things too.

Sometimes, it's easier for me to deal with the tragedies in life than the celebrations. When something good happens and I feel a pure, uplifting sensation, I don't always know how to respond. Why are we more used to feeling bad than feeling good? Know that whatever good is happening right now, it is time for that too. Welcome it in and embrace it. You have worked hard, and you deserve it.

DAY 202

I used to think people who didn't care about material possessions or getting ahead were crazy. I had no idea how to be motivated or inspired without the promise of gain or status. Yoga has taught me that pursuing the path of love and selflessness is more powerful than any worldly goods. Being on the path of yoga does not mean we can't achieve wealth, abundance, status, or fame if that is what is meant for us. When we let go of the belief that a material possession or ego-inflating promise will satisfy us, we are able to be fulfilled, whole, and complete all on our own. We stand on our own two feet, grounded in our truth no matter what the world brings or doesn't bring. We are not lured by false promises or shiny objects that only provide temporary comfort.

So many of our life choices are based on the illusion of what will bring us joy and peace. Your joy is inside you. Your access to peace is right here—right now. There is nothing you could attain that would bring you these qualities that you crave. Your practice of self-forgiveness teaches you to forgive. Your practice of self-compassion teaches you to understand. Your practice delivers gifts you once may have thought were impossible without material gain. We have been duped into thinking collecting things, people, and desires will end our suffering. Follow the advice from Swami Kripalu and "be a fool when confronted with worldly desires. That means being ignorant of their charms."[44] Remember that happiness is not found outside us but within.

....
44. Levitt, *Pilgrim of Love*, 111.

DAY 203

Sometimes, a physical injury or illness affects our ability to practice the way we are used to. This doesn't mean we have lost our practice or that we are unable to continue practicing. Whatever your practice looks like *is* the practice. Shortly after completing my yoga teacher training, I injured my shoulder and was unable to do several yoga postures until it healed. When I tried to hurry my healing by forcing my body into postures, my shoulder cried out in pain. We get attached to our practice like anything else. When our practice stops bolstering our ego, we feel like we are not good enough. We fear that if we skip meditating that day, we will never recover. We fear that if we do not complete our postures just like we always have, we will stop learning and growing. Physical limitations are humbling, and they do not prevent us from practicing yoga. In fact, if our mind is disturbed by a disruption to our practice, it is a great lesson in non-attachment. Why are we attached to what our practice should look like? Why is it so hard to meet ourselves where we are?

Life can get in the way of our practice as well. Jobs, children, family, and other responsibilities can all affect what our practice looks like. I can get so frustrated when the kids need me, when the dog needs me, or when there are other interruptions to my practice. Again, my ego clings to the way I want something to be instead of the way something is. Humility, kindness, understanding, and compassion are excellent qualities to welcome in when we are unsatisfied with our practice.

DAY 204

I lay on the bathroom floor and sobbed onto cold tile. I sobbed for every single failure, every single misstep, and every single wrong turn and bad decision that brought me here—divorced, addicted, and alone. At once, my world crashed in on me, and I knew I wouldn't be able to get back up without making a serious change. When I asked how this happened, my therapist said, "With addiction, it takes a perfect storm." Her sentence slammed into my chest like a boat crashing against a rocky shore. The cracks in my heart swelled with tender awareness and raw exposure. I couldn't be an alcoholic. Alcoholics were something else; they were someone who didn't look like me.

I wanted everything to go away, so I kept trying to date men after my divorce. I kept trying to drink. Ignore the pain. Replace the guy. Betray myself. I had no idea who I would be without my marriage. I got married because it was what people do. Plus, I wanted to feel complete.

Our path often chooses us. We can fight it or embrace it, but lessons will find us, and in my case, I had to really hit bottom in order to be jarred awake. A woman in recovery meetings used to say, "Let go or be dragged." In the beginning, I was dragged, desperate, and unconvinced. Thank goodness for that day I sobbed on the bathroom floor. The life I thought would fulfill me was full of holes and illusion. Stepping into the unknown has led to a permanent peace inside my body and an acceptance of myself that is not contingent on anyone else. Some things are easy to let go. Some are catastrophic. Those big ones are your saviors in disguise and the ones you will never regret.

DAY 205

At some point during my healing journey, the thought crossed my mind that I could stop trying so hard. I mouthed the words *"I accept myself as I am,"* and it felt as if a lump the size of a walnut, right below my rib cage, suddenly burst open. A warm, calming liquid poured throughout my abdomen and up inside my throat. Since then, I've stopped asking myself, *"What's wrong with me?"* And replaced it with: *"This is who I am."*

The mind-body connection is real, which is why physical manifestations can both be caused and healed by our thoughts. For whatever reason, my body reacted this way to my mind deciding to practice self-acceptance. I was present and aware enough in my body to notice the sensation. It really felt like a stone or nut cracking open and flowing out. Our bodies heal and let go when we give them permission.

Give yourself permission to let go. Often, we won't let go until something gets really bad and we hit some sort of bottom. When we can't take it anymore, when we have endured enough pain, we finally decide we might be able to ease up a bit. Your life doesn't have to fall apart in order to practice ungrasping. How badly do you want to keep trying so hard? How much do you want to suffer? Accepting yourself as you are today is a huge step in letting go and opening up to a brighter future.

DAY 206

Once we decide to let go, it's almost ridiculously simple. We spend most of our time worrying about letting go, resisting letting go, and being overall stubborn and fearful. But once we do, once we make the change that our heart knew was necessary, we feel a little lighter. We feel relief. Consider a time when you had trouble letting something go, but then, after you did, you felt immediately better. When you decided to quit your old job for a new one, an easy feeling came over you. When you told someone the relationship just wasn't working out anymore, you felt freer. Sometimes, when we let go, our body confirms for us that it is right. Of course we may second-guess ourselves afterward. When we have a challenge at our new job, we might long for the old one. But these feelings of looking back are fleeting, and we know that overall our decision was in our best interest.

If there is a weight you have been dragging around, it is possible to let go at once and without telling anyone. This weight can be a belief you hold about yourself, or it can be a life decision. Letting go requires no effort and no parade as an exit. Imagine it like a leaf falling from a tree with no sound and no one even watching. Now, if you could just let go.

DAY 207

Our material possessions provide much comfort, joy, and contentment. Meaningful objects are tied to our emotions, which is why it is difficult to imagine parting with them. The practice of aparigraha does not ask us to be rid of all possessions, but we can ask ourselves important questions concerning the role of our stuff.

You may collect meaningful objects from trips. The artwork in your home holds memories. Special gifts bring feelings of love. An important purchase makes you feel pride. Material possessions are meaningful as long we are not confusing the joy they bring with attachment. What if they went away? Would you still hold the same joy, pride, memory, contentment, and security? Or would the absence of that possession control your mood or your feelings of safety? This is when we know that a possession owns us instead of the other way around. If being rid of the object brings fear, examine that.

One way to practice nonattachment is to appreciate our possessions in the present moment while acknowledging we may not always have them. Be grateful for your pillow and warm bed at night. Enjoy your tea out of your favorite mug and be grateful for its role in your morning routine. Life changes. Nothing is guaranteed. Instead of taking the objects in your life for granted, appreciate them without letting them control you or your mood. With gratitude, accept objects for what they are—a comfort, an indulgence, and a way to make our life easier. An object does not define who we are, and we would be the same person, have the same memories, and hold the same accomplishments with or without these possessions.

DAY 208
Observing the Breath

Observing the breath while holding it, either at the top of the inhale or the bottom of the exhale, teaches us a lot about letting go and trusting that the next breath will always arrive. Holding the breath is also an interesting practice to see where we are familiar, either in feelings of emptiness or sensations of being full.

To practice, *inhale smoothly for four to five counts. Fill the belly, ribs, and upper chest, not by force but with a long, even inhale. Then hold. Stay holding the breath for several counts and observe what happens. Does the mind get restless? Does fear arrive? Watch the sensation of craving for the exhale.*

You can also practice holding the breath at the bottom of the exhale. To do this, *exhale completely, and then hold the breath at the bottom of the exhale. Observe the sensation of emptiness. What does it feel like to be empty? Do sensations of fear or restlessness arrive, or are the sensations a little different?*

While holding the breath full, we learn a lot about our reactions to craving and lack. Knowing you will be holding the breath, for example, do you take an extra deep inhale? Do you make sure you will have enough air to hold for a longer time? Likewise, what is your experience squeezing out the exhale and allowing yourself to be empty? Some people are more comfortable holding the inhale; they're more familiar with the sensation of being full. Others are more comfortable at the bottom of the exhale; they're more familiar with the sensation of emptiness. Notice what arrives for you.

DAY 209

I have a terrible habit of trying to do it all. At one point in my life, I was running a business, teaching at a college, teaching yoga, and writing my first book. I was also raising two young boys. I felt like I was going through the motions but not really excelling. Everything got a small part of me, and I was heavy with guilt when I couldn't give my all. A friend suggested letting something go. I winced. I feared letting the wrong thing go and of losing income and stability. I felt that the more I did, the safer we would all be.

Like so often happens, the Universe stepped in to do for me what I could not do for myself. The college I worked for closed their campus, and I lost my teaching job. Shortly after, COVID-19 closed the yoga studios. I started teaching through Facebook during quarantine, thinking it would be temporary. After several months, now home all day with my boys, I realized the world was not going back to the way it used to be anytime soon. One day, we were living in a certain reality. The next day, it felt as if the whole world changed.

Being let go from my teaching position was a gift in disguise. I started my online yoga membership, and it has been the perfect blend of my teaching, writing, and yoga. I can be present for my job, my boys, and myself. Had I kept all the jobs—all the roles as a safety net—I never would have moved forward. Sometimes, the path needs to be shown to us. Pay attention.

DAY 210

Disappointment often comes after an expectation has not been met. We hold expectations around so many things: how we want people to act, how we want an experience to make us feel, and how we want something to turn out. Our expectations of people can make us blame them for our disappointment instead of looking at our own attachments. Of course people will disappoint us, but if we are constantly requiring others to behave a certain way in order to fulfill us, no one will live up to our expectations. People are not robots. We all have changing emotions, moods, and tendencies. It's not someone else's responsibility to always know what we need or always act the way we need them to. It's also not realistic to expect that someone will act the same way every single time or that our experience with them will never change or shift.

Healthy relationships have deep amounts of respect, understanding, and individuality. We practice being fulfilled from within so we are not unfairly relying on others to do it for us. We learn to let go of so many expectations and instead enjoy and accept the person as they are. If we are always demanding that our expectations be met, whether it's by a person, a place, or an experience, we are not able to be present. We are bogged down by the idea we have in our mind or the story we are telling ourselves, and we cannot even see what's happening right here, right now. Let go of expectations, and you will be less disappointed. You will also be given the gift of knowing someone as they are instead of what you want them to be.

DAY 211

If we accept impermanence as a part of life, we can be more present and alive for what is. It's natural to attach to good feelings and experiences and never want them to end. We chase the good feelings and try to re-create them. Just because something doesn't provide the same experience or emotion as it did before, doesn't necessarily point to anything being wrong.

A delicious meal is a wonderful feeling. Senses wake up. We feel content and pleasured. We feel nourished and alive. I went to a new restaurant and ordered a seared tomato and mozzarella cheese appetizer. It came with grilled toast drizzled in the sweetest balsamic glaze. Tender artichoke hearts sat nestled on top of an almond spread. When I took the perfect bite of bread, tomato, artichoke, and almond spread, I couldn't contain my enthusiasm. I indulged in the entire plate. A few months later, I went back to the restaurant with a friend and went on and on about this amazing dish. The meal arrived—the exact same recipe on an identical plate. I took my first bite. But I was underwhelmed. *Was there the exact same amount of balsamic drizzle? Was the cheese as soft?* I tried to re-create my experience, and nothing was different about the food; I was different. Not only had I built this food up in my head but I expected the same ecstatic experience as the first time. I still enjoyed it, but by chasing the same feeling, I dimmed my current experience. Impermanence applies to all experiences, emotions, and good feelings. Not much can be re-created, so enjoy those moments of pure pleasure, and accept them for what they are.

DAY 212
Double Pigeon Pose

Double pigeon pose, also called fire log pose, is an excellent hip opener. With regular practice, you'll notice quick progress.

> *Begin seated. Bend one leg and keep your foot away from your seat, trying to make your shin parallel to the edge of your mat. Stack your other leg on top, with the ankle on top of the knee and the knee on top of the ankle. The idea is that both shins are "stacked" like logs.*

I struggle in this pose. My knees never rest all the way down like neatly stacked logs. They are more like unruly kindling trying to leap away from the fire. If your top leg angles up, don't worry. Keep the foot over the opposite knee and notice when the sensation in your hips becomes strong. Feel into your body's alignment to a place where you can sit and breathe without the discomfort being too much of a distraction. Let the sensation be your guide. Breathe.

Because of our lifestyle of sitting, it's common for the hips to get tight and sore. We also hold a lot of emotion in our hips. The ache in my hips while in fire log pose is steady and persistent. My questions are always, "What am I holding in there? What am I refusing to let go?"

That's the deep work and the beauty of yoga; we don't have to know what we are holding in order to let it go. Anything that comes up has a purpose, and when we release physical discomfort or pain, we also cleanse and release something emotional. Something has shifted. Something that used to be is no longer.

DAY 213

Yoga is a path of inquiry that leads us to self-awareness. Yoga is not a goal, prescription, or answer. Yoga is inside you, so you get to ask your questions and choose what's best. You get to be the creator of your life by cultivating a loving relationship with your body and your soul so you can operate from a place of self-compassion and truth instead of what everyone else wants from you. You get to determine the path of your life. You get to determine how you spend your time each day.

Start saying *no* to things you don't want to do. Start saying *yes* to things that light you up. This is not to say we should only have fun and never work; work is rewarding and fulfilling when we're utilizing our skills and talents.

What is holding you back from spending each day doing what you love? Fear? Obligation? Responsibility?

It is not selfish to create the life of your dreams. It is not selfish to let go of things you don't like. Maybe you used to like a hobby or profession, but now you don't, and that is okay. Maybe there is a new skill you want to learn. Maybe you have been meeting the same group of people every Monday night for cocktails, and you're no longer into it. Your time is precious. There is always this one day; spend it wisely.

DAY 214

Aparigraha is a lifelong practice that will come up again and again during your journey. We let something go, and it inevitably resurfaces. We must let go again. In our world of striving, collecting, amassing, and achievement, there is no lack of opportunity to practice letting go. Daily we are pummeled with ads and products that promise to fulfill us. Businesses point out our supposed voids, and we attempt to fill them. We become afraid to rid ourselves of anything for fear we won't recover or fear of missing out. We become tied to our things. Actually, we become imprisoned by them.

My hope is that you have softened around this idea of ungrasping and experienced some of the relief that arrives when we release our grip. I hope you have become more observant and less willful. I hope you have thrown out what is heavy and cumbersome. I hope you have let go in order to rise to the next venture.

Give yourself some space to think about how far you've come and what has been revealed. Letting go is a process accomplished through awareness, trust, and, finally, surrender. If you've come to a realization about something you would like to let go, such as a belief, a behavior, a pattern, or an emotion, you have already begun the process of letting go. This practice has been deep, insightful, and challenging. Breathe in. Breathe out. Breathe in, trust yourself, and as you exhale, sigh out a long and loud, "*I let go.*"

PRACTICE 8
Surrender (Ishvara Pranidhana)

In Patanjali's Yoga Sutras, the practice of *ishvara pranidhana* means "to surrender to the infinite, or all-knowing." It also states offering all our actions to the "Supreme God."[45] Surrender is the last of Patanjali's five niyamas, yoga's ethical practices for living a peaceful and fulfilled life. It's important to clarify that *God*, or *all-knowing*, as it translates from yoga, has nothing to do with religion. The infinite beyond signifies a greater energy outside us. This energy can be God, nature, or collective consciousness. Ishvara pranidhana has to do with connecting to our higher Self instead of our ego. It means walking with the Divine, being in flow with the energy of the Universe, and offering our actions in favor of the greater good. Surrender means living a life of service, which includes taking care of our own spirituality. We practice letting go of our self-will and surrendering to something outside of ourselves for answers, for strength, and for discovering our destiny.

....

45. Satchidananda, *The Yoga Sutras of Patanjali*, 37–38.

DAY 215

When have you surrendered? Usually, to enact ishvara pranidhana, we must be up against a wall. Rarely do we relinquish control until we absolutely have to. We often do it only when we feel there is no other way. Our ego holds on tightly to our beliefs about the world and our beliefs about ourselves. These are beliefs about how others should act and behave and what our life should look like. Surrender is hard! What if we surrender and we don't get the outcome we want? What if we let go and lose all control? We want to stay comfortable, even when it is limiting. We have trouble believing that by surrendering fully, by opening to all possibilities, both good and bad, we will actually be given exactly what we need.

I like to think of surrendering as a willingness to rely on something outside myself—something I cannot see or touch. An example of this is relying on my heart or my intuition to point me in the right direction. I rely on my higher Self and the sensations in my body to steer me. It may not be practical, but I rarely regret it.

When have you surrendered? When have you relied on something outside your thinking mind in order to make a change or a choice? When have you felt compelled to do something or not do something without a logical reason? When have you just "felt" it?

DAY 216

A simple (yet sometimes difficult) way to start practicing surrender is to lead with your heart. Try this during your yoga practice, and consider the poses as opportunities to move into your body and out of your mind. Notice if your body intuitively knows what it needs. Stop worrying about the sequence or the pose, and let your heart be your guide. Trust that listening to your heart is okay; you are not doing anything wrong.

Practice leading with your heart in life situations. Tune in to the deeper part of yourself before you have an important conversation, before you start your workday, or before you make a big decision. Notice if you can sense what "feels" right.

Tuning in connects us with the energy within ourselves and the energy of the Universe. We allow for awareness of something greater than ourselves—something we cannot name, see, or touch. The times I have surrendered and let go of control have ultimately led me to places I never would have considered or chosen for myself. The times I have surrendered have taught me that I can let go, and it will be okay. In fact, the times I have surrendered have led to outcomes much better than what I would have chosen for myself.

DAY 217

According to the Sutras, "Ishvara Pranidhana is a life of dedication, of offering everything to God or to humanity."[46] A life of dedication and service does not mean we cannot have fun, we cannot go after our dreams, or we need to give away all our money to charity. A life of dedication and service means we follow the path that helps everyone—ourselves and all others. How do we know what this path is? The path of service looks different for everyone. Maybe you are a parent or caregiver. Maybe you volunteer your time or donate financially. Professions are service and so are creative pursuits. When we ask what we can offer—instead of how we can profit—we are already surrendering. Sharing our gifts with others is why we are here. We are meant to bring our gifts and our talents forth so we can be of service to others and be fulfilled within. Surrendering is a form of detachment. By offering ourselves to humanity, we are automatically connected to the greater good. We are no longer bound by possessions or the mental chattering of the ego. We have nothing to worry about because we know that as long as we keep living with an attitude of service, we will continually be at peace and fulfilled.

....
46. Satchidananda, *The Yoga Sutras of Patanjali*, 141.

DAY 218

To live a peaceful life, we don't have to control other people. We don't have to fix other people. We don't even have to fix ourselves. Part of the practice of surrender means we accept.

Can you, right in this moment, accept yourself as you are? Do you think you are perfect today? Or would you rather lose fifteen pounds, get a certain job, pass a test, make an amount of money, reach a personal goal ... and *then*, then you will be perfect?

We fear accepting ourselves and others because we think it means we won't reach our goals or we will stop caring. We won't lose the weight, get a promotion, or achieve what we want. The other person, whom we want to change, will never change unless we tell them to or show them how. Acceptance of something in the moment does not mean settling for it to always be that way. We can still have goals, dreams, pursuits, and lessons. We can still nurture and deepen relationships. We can set boundaries and tell others how we feel. Surrender is not giving up or allowing an enemy to win. Surrender allows something else to step in—something much more powerful than us. Surrender allows for grace, for compassion, and for radical acceptance. Rather than punish yourself or refuse to accept where you are right now, know that when you surrender to something outside of yourself, when you trust in the greater good, you are pointed in the right direction. People and opportunities show up, you know what to do next, and you start to feel more at peace as you make progress.

DAY 219

I always thought life was a conquest. It was something to win at. Something to get an A+ on. I just wanted to do everything right. In the process, I never surrendered. Surrendering would indicate failure or needing help. I didn't want anyone to see me sweat. *Wasn't that a badge of honor or something?* It turns out, you get no points for being perfect or being alone. I felt lonely, purposeless, and lost. I had it backward. Instead of asking what I could offer, I asked what would make me feel better. My dear friend Kate texted me one day just before I quit drinking. She wrote, "Heal yourself, so you can help others heal."

I had no idea what her words meant, but they pelted at my heart like a soft spring rain on still frozen earth. It never occurred to me that my pain could help others. It never occurred to me that my pain was anything other than punishment and my burden to bear. Her words brought me a moment of surrender. I opened to the possibility that I had a problem and that I would have to do something about it. I opened to the possibility that if I trusted in something outside of myself, if I surrendered to what was happening, I would be shown the way. Peace and knowing enter each time we surrender and each time we accept where we are. You do not have to do any of this on your own. You get no points for being an island or being perfect at life. Your path can help someone else on theirs, so be open to letting someone or something else show you the way.

DAY 220

Anything we hold space for will show up on our mat. Since we are thinking about surrender, you can recognize qualities of surrender during your yoga practice or meditation. Some qualities of surrender are trust, observation, offering and receiving, nonattachment, and presence. Begin by welcoming these qualities of surrender into your yoga practice and into your day. Move through postures with an intention of offering. Where does your heart go and what comes up? Invite trust into your practice, possibly during a balance pose or a pose you tend to avoid. Let go of expectations for your practice, and let it be perfect exactly the way it is. Notice how bringing surrender into your yoga practice changes your approach to postures or your overall experience.

Other ways to practice surrender are through daily rituals or activities. During meditation, set an intention to receive. Close your eyes and open your palms. Be open to healing, inspiration, or possibility. When faced with a dilemma, ask your gut or your heart what it thinks. Become more skilled at tuning in to and answering your body. Test it out in life choices. Practice a moving devotion, which means you are doing something but also surrendering to the body and the motion. Moving devotions can be done with repetitive activities like knitting, cooking, or walking. Complete a symbolic ritual in order to surrender something to the Divine. Write what you would like to surrender on a piece of paper, such as a person, a relationship, a difficult situation, or a personal character trait. You can burn the paper or tuck it in a box, surrendering the outcome and trusting you will be shown the way.

DAY 221

In my experience, peace, faith, and love (all the big ones) have been shown to me in moments that are not filled with people, tasks, or even successes. Faith that everything is always as it should be, past and present, arrives when I am still. It arrives when outside noises have been quelled and my breath is slow and even. In stillness, I see more clearly. In the quiet, I sense that something bigger is happening, and I am not doing it.

A sense of being held is often all we need to step out of our inner turmoil and into unwavering belief. Faith does not depend on an outcome or anything exterior to look a certain way. Faith is often the opposite. It is belief despite how something appears. Faith can be in a higher power or something outside of you. Faith can also be in yourself. Faith is moving forward without knowing what will happen next. Faith is believing that however you proceed, the result will be good for you and for everyone.

It's very easy to let setbacks weaken our faith. We have a bad day. We wonder if all this belief and trust is worth anything. Humans move through life in a certain amount of pain and ignorance. We can't see the big picture, and we want to know the reasons why. But in life, we don't get all the answers. We only see the next few steps in front of us. Luckily, signs and synchronicities, such as a helpful person, a repetitious word, or a chance encounter, show up. I think the Universe gives these signs because it knows we need a little reassurance.

DAY 222

Most of the time, we can manage just fine with a certain amount of stress, a bit of overwhelm, and an awareness of the unknown. But sometimes, the path gets really unbearable. We feel ourselves slipping off the beam, and we wonder if we have missed something. How do we resume our faith when we have lost it? What do we do when hopelessness and despair take over? Some people pray. Some people meditate. Some people go for a walk. In any of these situations, the commonality is in the "not doing." The moment we throw our hands in the air, something has just shifted. We have replaced our control with surrender.

During times of hopelessness and despair, the present moment is your friend. All of your senses and what you can observe in this moment are your relief. Watch and observe. Watch your own feelings. Watch something in nature. Watch your child, watch your pet, or listen to the rain fall on your windows. Glimpse the beauty that exists in one single moment, and stop doing whatever you think you should be doing.

Stop trying to figure out the plan. Stop trying to master the Universe. When I actually stop and say to myself, *"I can't do this anymore,"* something miraculously shifts. My footing becomes immediately firmer. In the letting go and in the permission to "not do," I feel comforted. When all faith is lost, surrender.

DAY 223

We get in our own way. We are so busy orchestrating for the sake of ourselves and others, we cannot see the opportunities actually meant for us. We go after something only to be disappointed, but if we would have surrendered our intention in the first place, we may have recognized the hidden gift that lies in every single experience. Trust that everything is in your favor. Once you do, there are few moments to be disappointed.

It's hard to imagine the ease and peace we would experience if we moved through life with complete trust in a greater good. It doesn't matter if you believe in a god or in humanity. We still think we know what's best. Guess what? The greater plan is much, much, *much* better than yours. You are upset that your relationship ended, the rejection letter arrived, or the car got dented. Meanwhile, the Universe has something brilliant in store for you, and these incidents are necessary to get you there. We don't know why, and that's okay. Just like we can observe physical discomfort during a yoga pose with an attitude of nonjudgment, we can try doing the same in life. Things don't have to be good or bad. They just are. It doesn't mean we should stop going after things or stop trying. Keep looking for the perfect partner. Keep sending submissions or applying for jobs. When the answer is no, trust that the particular opportunity was not best for you, and the right one is on its way.

DAY 224

Life is not about trying to master the art of control and manipulation. Even when we get what we want, it never satisfies. Life is about learning to surrender so we can be at ease in the moment. Easeful moments of presence add up, and we reach our potential anyway without the anxiety of our own fears and doubts. Here are some journal prompts that will provide relief around a situation that is causing discomfort, anxiety, or fear.

First, choose a difficult situation; it can be work-related, body-related, relationship-related, or a character trait.

Then explore these prompts in your journal:

+ Where is my ego showing up in this situation? For example, where am I grabbing at control? What does my handling of the situation look like right now?
+ What qualities of surrender can I enact? What would it look like to trust, to let go of the outcome, or to offer instead of expect?
+ What rituals of surrender can I do around this situation? Can I practice yoga, go for a walk, do a symbolic burning, or something else?

After writing, put some of your thoughts into practice. Do one thing as an act of surrender toward your current circumstance. See if you feel more trusting and at ease.

DAY 225

The idea of surrender goes against many beliefs in modern society such as never giving up, pushing through at all costs, and, in general, striving. We have been fed the idea of action in order to produce results, and surrender feels very weak and passive in comparison.

Surrender does not mean admitting defeat or giving up. Surrender also doesn't mean we stop taking action. Surrender is a loving and intentional way to offer something up to the greater good. We can release outcome and our own expectation in order to receive all the gifts that are meant for us. Surrender is a practice in accepting that we don't know all the answers. We turn our problem over to fate, a higher power, or our own energy and consciousness. Surrender is actually very brave. At a low point and after so much striving, we finally relinquish control.

Surrender does not have to be practiced only when we are at rock bottom. Often, we need to be pushed to such a level of suffering and discomfort in order to let go. But there are many ways you can surrender in your everyday life and undo the core belief that in order to get what we want, we must push, force, and strive. We can accomplish our tasks but with an attitude of surrender. I can have a very busy day yet be completely unproductive. Likewise, I can have a very productive day with amazing outcomes while not trying so hard. Notice if your frantic busyness or fearful pushing yields beneficial results. Also pay attention to when you are moving in "flow" with the Universe, and things seem to get accomplished without so much of your energy.

DAY 226

Surrender allows some of the best parts of us, such as presence, joy, humility, acceptance, forgiveness, and gratitude, to rise to the surface. When we surrender, we release the burden of trying to meet the ego's demands. Surrender brings us out of ourselves and into belonging. No longer are we alone in our efforts. We let go and remain open to anything that arrives. We decide to stop fighting for our own benefit and live as a part of the greater community. My mother-in-law and I didn't get along well at first. It turns out, we were eerily similar, but we both fought for our role in the family. Our egos banged into one another whenever we felt encroached on. In reality, we did not have to compete at all. Sometimes, we are bothered by someone and are unaware of the reasons behind it. When we seek to understand others and see them as ourselves, we create connection. The ego wants to keep us separate so we will stay stuck in blaming and wanting the other person to change in order to meet our requirements. Through surrender, we drop the ego and begin to see our situation with the eyes of the compassionate Self. There is always enough love—love for parents, for children, and for friends. We can expand our view and our hearts and welcome everyone in. In return, we will receive more of the love we actually crave, and the fear of not belonging will drift away like a passing storm. The memories I have with my mother-in-law—the times we were fully present for each other and not in competition—are moments I cherish and long to have back.

DAY 227

Often, we are brought to a place of surrender because the practice is exactly what we need. We arrive kicking and screaming about something that is not going our way, and we have forgotten the power of rest and release. We have forgotten the power in the force greater than us. Consider the delicious rest in child's pose or the sweet feeling of completion in shavasana. These moments prove enlightening and necessary for your practice. Life is the same; we need some moments of pause and of rest. If you feel like you are flailing, your footing can find solid ground in the surrender. We become humble, we become faithful, and we abide. We sit still for the first time in a long time, and after the initial resistance, we settle in and think, "Wow, this feels pretty good." Surrender gives you a break. When we surrender to an energy outside ourselves, when we bow our forehead to the mat or lie on our back wide open, we welcome in wisdom from our own heart. We welcome in whispers from the Divine. Our body at rest signals an offering, not only of the body but of our spirit, to receive guidance, love, or healing. *Take this. Take this from me because I can't.* These are powerful words. Even saying them out loud brings an ache in my chest and wetness at my eyes. No matter what you believe in, a part of you needs to offer these words and this intention. We all meet a breaking point, and surrendering turns our struggles over or at least sets them down. Allow something else to take over, even for a moment, so you can rest and be refreshed.

DAY 228
Container Meditation

Seated or lying down, take a few letting-go breaths, inhaling through the nose and exhaling out the mouth. Do this at least three times. Allow your body and the muscles to relax. Close your eyes and let the face soften—the eyelids, the cheeks, and your jaw. Observe your breath. Imagine a box or container. Let the container look like anything you want. It can be a vessel you already own or something completely made up. The box can have a lid or be of any shape. Now, think of a conflict or current struggle. Hold the conflict in your mind, and then, with care, place that struggle in the container. Think of another conflict, and place that in the container. One by one, let every disturbance arrive, and place each one in the container. Continue until the container holds everything, all your heaviness, all your burdens, and all the things you want to change. Observe your body now that all your desires and conflicts are inside the box. Now, imagine a beam of light pouring down from the sky and shining directly on your container. The container starts to move, carried up by the light, and it is eventually out of sight.

Once the container is carried away, how do you feel? Are there items you placed in the box you now wish you hadn't? Are you relieved that all of them are gone? Let the image of the container go, and place a hand on your heart. Say to yourself or out loud, "*I am safe.*" "*I am protected.*" "*It is safe to let these things go.*"

You can do this meditation again and again, noticing if letting go of certain items in the container gets any easier.

DAY 229

Maybe we don't have as much control as we think, or at least not where we try to exert it. Instead of trying to make life, people, and circumstances bend to meet our desires, we can consider where we might change. The serenity prayer offers that we first accept that which is out of our control. "Grant me the serenity to accept the things I cannot change, courage to change the things I can, and wisdom to know the difference."[47]

Courage is suggested as a next step; change takes courage because it means getting out of our comfort zone, challenging our beliefs, and actively engaging in a new behavior. Courage to change might look like standing up for ourselves or ending a vicious cycle. Courage to change might look as simple and as grueling as quietly walking away. Courage is admitting our feelings and following our intuition. Courage is making necessary but difficult choices.

Finally, the prayer asks for wisdom. Without an awareness of what is within our control and what isn't, we will fight, struggle, and wonder why nothing is changing. So, what can we control? Not a lot and yet so much. While we can't control death or illness, we can certainly adopt a healthy diet and lifestyle. While we can't change another person, we can lead by example. While we can't force an outcome, we can move toward a destination. The prayer's promise is serenity and matches the promise of yoga—the promise of peace and contentment through awareness, acceptance, and continued practice.

....
47. Niebuhr, "The Serenity Prayer and Twelve Step Recovery."

DAY 230

Surrender to people with whom you disagree. I believe that everyone is doing their best all the time, and we have no idea how someone's experiences have shaped them. Think of all the ways you operate with an amount of unawareness. Everyone else is unaware as well. We don't necessarily know why we feel frustrated or out of sorts one day. It could be circumstantial, but it could also be a number of old wounds or buried emotions. What comes out on the surface is never the whole story. Doing the work to peel away layers of a lifetime of experience takes practice, dedication, and support—but the desire to change needs to come from within. Many people are perfectly fine with their behaviors and choices. We may think we know what is best for them, but they have their own path, and we have ours. We cannot force people to look at themselves.

Furthermore, it's possible to avoid our own problems by trying to fix and save others. We can support someone by listening but not necessarily lending advice. Being a helper is a fabulous way to not look at ourselves. Helping may be a desire for purpose or usefulness. If you are a helper, ask yourself what is being fulfilled by trying to fix other people. Are there other ways you might find purpose or build self-worth? Being there for those we love comes from a very good place. Healing and growing from within and demonstrating that we can be fulfilled without relying on someone else is the most helpful gift we can give to those we care about.

DAY 231

Jai Bhagwan is Sanskrit for "victory to spirit." The phrase is used as both a greeting and a blessing while acknowledging a force greater than ourselves. "Victory to spirit" means we trust spirit's plan over our own because we know it is better, grander, and more beneficial for all. Sanskrit words have multiple definitions. *Jai* means "victory." And *Bhagwan* means "spirit" as well as "prosperous." Saying *Jai Bhagwan* at the end of a yoga practice or in response to someone's news means, "I wish for the greatest good and the best outcome for all." The phrase acknowledges our heartfelt hope that all turns out well with the understanding that we don't know what "good" really looks like.

Surrendering to spirit means you release your expectation. Surrendering does not mean you sit back and watch the Universe unfold perfectly in front of you. You still have to put in a lot of effort and possibly trial and error in order to dance with the Divine. Your specific goals playing out exactly as you see them might not be the intended path. But if we all act on the faith that no matter what happens, no matter how painful or ugly life gets, there is something bigger conspiring toward the greatest good for all, then we can at least move forward with love in our hearts instead of turmoil and judgment. We can work toward our desires without fearing whether they will manifest. We can take solace that even when things appear to be going not as planned, all of it is in our favor. It just doesn't look the way we expected. Continually keeping the phrase *Jai Bhagwan* at the center of our intention ensures victory for all.

DAY 232

Did you know the "greater good" also includes you? Just because something isn't how you want it, doesn't mean the Universe has forgotten about you. You are deserving, worthy, and part of the grand plan. Achieving the greatest good for all might mean you have to do something you don't want to do. The greatest good for all might mean you have to leave something you're not ready to let go. The greatest good for all might mean you have to change something you're currently afraid to change.

Take a minute and ask yourself, *"What do I need to hear right now?"* Your heart already knows. Your wise intuition tells you the next right move. You don't have to resist your inner voice just because it's telling you something you don't want to hear. There's a difference between talking yourself out of something hard and following your gut. When you follow your gut, you feel at peace, even if it's difficult to hear. Looking back, anytime we have made a hard decision, we are usually able to pinpoint the moment we knew. We probably resisted for a while and life got worse. But eventually, we listened to the inner voice that told us the answer a long time ago. Listening to the wise inner voice is like flowing with the Universe. It's like saying to your higher Self, *"Fine! I'll do it! I don't want to, but I will. So, you better show me something good."* Play with the Universe; call it out.

It's going to be okay. The Universe will not disappoint. It might be painful at first, but you will come out better on the other side. Yes, the greater good includes you.

DAY 233

When I attended my monthlong teacher training at Kripalu, I was immersed in deep inner work. Of course my surroundings were beautiful and indulgent. My daily schedule was planned. My meals were prepared. My room was cleaned. I had no chores or children or job. Yet there were days that were extremely difficult and much more emotionally challenging than anything at home. Friends would email and ask, "How are you enjoying your retreat?" as if I was on vacation. I couldn't describe the roller coaster of my experience because I was doing yoga, meditating, and spending time in nature—what could be difficult? We expect that our new yoga and meditation routine will make us feel better, so it is a bit jarring when we start to feel worse.

But any problems arriving are not signs of a misstep; they are a sign that your practice is working. Without the distraction of outside people or events, you are finally with yourself, and opportunities to heal are bursting to the forefront. One day, I had a particularly painful memory—a flashback of childhood trauma. I thought I may need to give up. This seemed too much. I wrote in my journal and trusted I was safe. I *felt* safe. I knew that if I got too uncomfortable, I could stop at any point. Just like a pose, we know how long to stay and when to get out. This is the practice of compassionate self-observation. It is trusting that you are safe to stay and trusting you will know when it is too much.

DAY 234

Have you ever thought of something and it immediately happened? Examples from my own life would be when a friend popped into my mind and she called right then. There was also the time I asked for clarity about my house, which wouldn't sell, and I got a text from someone who wanted to rent it. And then there was the time I declared to the Universe, "*I need a job.*" I emailed a woman about teaching opportunities, and she called me five minutes later to tell me someone had just quit.

We are always sending arrows of intention into the Universe, and the arrows are designed to land where they were aimed—that's physics. Of course something could throw our arrow off course. Sometimes, it is the wind or an element out of our control. Sometimes, it is our own doubts and meddling. If the arrow is our intention, we have to let it go and trust where it will land. Imagine you take aim, pull back on your bow, and release. Then imagine you run after the arrow in order to make sure it's okay. Imagine you babysit your arrow after it leaves your fingertips. We don't need to intervene with the arrow, but we do need to take action that supports our intention. Apply for the job. Apply for many jobs. Submit the essay. Go on the date. I challenge you to consider your beliefs around your intentions. Have faith that nothing is out of reach, and nothing is too far away. Your aim could be realized immediately or over time and in a way you hadn't considered. Be patient but steadfast. The arrow is designed to hit its mark, and we are constantly in communication with the Universe.

DAY 235

During a yoga practice, arriving on the mat or meditation cushion is half the battle. We start by showing up. From there, seize the moment. Stretch yourself through every posture, move through resistance and doubt, and stay present and in tune with your body. Make your practice worthwhile, whether that looks like staying in child's pose or holding yourself upright for five more breaths. When you are immersed in the effort of the moment, you quiet the normal thinking of the mind. You do better, and insight is more available. Do not mindlessly move through the motions of the practice, thinking ahead to the next chore on your list. Be right there.

So is the case in life. Attention on your work, your play, and your routine brings contentment and makes the activity meaningful. The mind is what carries us away from the moment. The mind jumps us ahead to something yet to occur, and we have lost the present moment. Moments can be long or short, but every moment we truly show up for is essential to our being. When the moment ends, when we come down to our mat for shavasana, we acknowledge the effort is complete. Tired muscles point to our effort. No matter how our yoga practice went, we can rest easily in the fact that we showed up and gave everything we had. We touched the present moment and acknowledged our entire Self. When the effort is complete, acknowledge that as well and feel permission to let go.

DAY 236

Yoga, if you are seeking it, is above all a spiritual path. Yoga does not ask you to believe in anything in particular, but the practice of surrender asks that you turn your problems over to something outside yourself. Why? Turning something over connects us to the part of us that is universal love. It connects us to our truest, purest state and to the wisdom of collective consciousness. According to yoga, we are human and also divine. The practice of surrender helps us to feel less separate and more connected, whether that connection is to your higher Self, a god of your understanding, or all of humanity. Through surrender, we find union. We find purpose. Yoga has brought me closer to my understanding of Self than anything else I have done in my life. The physical practice of yoga connects me to my true feelings and helps me stay present with sensations. The spiritual practice of surrender reminds me I am not alone. This connection, this knowing I am not alone, is my source of unconditional love.

Both on your mat and in life, surrender. On an exhale, ungrip your toes and unclench your jaw. You don't have to try so hard. Letting go makes the posture more easeful and available. When life gives you pain or opportunities for growth, rely on your breath and your stillness to support you. Trust in the energy of love that exists outside of you. Know that you are unconditionally loved. Practice surrendering on your mat, and notice if a sensation of love or support arrives. This is all that is meant by surrendering outside yourself. Connect with that energy, which reminds you that you are not alone.

DAY 237

We all probably know the old philosophical question of "If a tree falls in the forest and no one is around to hear it, does it make a sound?" Today, this phrase could be replaced with "Until I google it, does it exist?" A look at our googling history could portray a pretty accurate depiction of our concerns. I've googled nearly everything that I want validation for. *How to know if I'm an alcoholic. Symptoms of depression. Signs your relationship is doomed.* One of my most recent searches was pretty telling: *How to just let go.* If you are wondering, google doesn't know the answer.

By the time I make it to that little box on my computer, I already know the answer. I know I am addicted. I know I am depressed. I know I'm in an unhealthy relationship. Radical acceptance is not passive. The first step toward any change is acceptance of the way things are. Acceptance doesn't mean we feel ready. We want to hide, and there are oh-so-many great hiding places—anger, isolation, food, substance, starvation, self-righteousness, rumination, gossip, lashing out, blame, and, of course, denial. Anything to avoid the unbearable squeeze of change. When something nags at you, pay attention. It might be time to surrender and accept. The longer we wait to make a change, the longer the inevitable will keep trying to get our attention. You don't have to wait. If you're sick of your life looking a certain way, you can surrender before it gets out of hand. Your heart always leads you to the best place, and you will be supported by the energy of love all along the way.

DAY 238
Open Awareness Meditation

An open awareness meditation is helpful when you have a particularly active mind, helping you to notice sensations without attaching. Do this exercise more than once and see how it changes. Meditation doesn't have to be rigid. Give yourself permission to explore a meditation that allows for all senses within your experience.

Begin by noticing the breath. Remember, you are observing and not forcing. There is nothing you need to change about the breath. Simply watch how it moves and feels. Focus your attention on the nostrils, breathing air in and out, or on your belly, expanding and contracting with breath. After watching your breath for a few moments, let your awareness travel to other sounds, smells, or sensations in the room. Maybe you hear a dog barking. Maybe there are children or people in the distance. Maybe raindrops are hitting the windows. Instead of trying to shut out these experiences or ignore them, allow all of the sensations to become part of your meditation. Observe how you can listen to the dog barking without attaching a narrative. Your mind might say, "Shoot, that dog is ruining my meditation!" But try not to let yourself worry or judge. The dog is not the problem. Your mind's story is preventing you from staying present. Notice the sound or distraction, and notice the next sound or sensation that arrives. Notice that all sensations pass through.

In a state of allowing and free from criticism, see how your meditation becomes a full experience of all that is present. Practice allowing without judgment during yoga so you can do the same in life.

DAY 239

Sun shines down on my outstretched arms as I stand strong in side warrior, back leg straight and sideways, front knee bent, thigh muscles rippling. The sand beneath my mat creates an unpredictable foundation. I wiggle my side-facing foot in deeply, trying to utilize the softness.

When we move from side warrior to warrior three, a balance on one leg, I am all of a sudden unsure. *Will I fall today? Tip at least?* When we let go, there is a moment of excitement while we also hold on for dear life. Gripping my toes fiercely into the sand, I try not to crumble as I lift my back leg off the ground. Immediately, the thigh muscles in my standing leg begin to shake. I recall scene after scene from my life when I've pretended to surrender while still clinging desperately to a self-fulfilling result. I will attempt the balance but only if I don't fall in front of the class. I will accept a failed relationship as long as I have another one to catch me. I will dive into the new adventure as long as there is a guarantee. I will offer my whole heart as long as it doesn't get broken. We surrender—but with safety nets.

Balancing in warrior three, I decide to give the pose everything I have. I loosen the grip of my toes in the sand and distribute my effort to my leg. I experience moments of floating while also wobbling. I surrender again and place effort in my core. When finished, I arrive in tadasana with both feet safely in the sand. With the pose and the effort complete, I breathe relief and let go.

DAY 240

We have ownership and responsibility over our life, but sometimes, we place too much stake in our level of control. As we have explored surrender, we have practiced letting go of outcomes and allowing grace to step in. We trust that what is meant for us will be delivered, and what is not meant for us will be removed. We may feel upset or unsure when we don't get what we want or when a person does not behave how we would like, but in the end, we are reminded of the dance between effort and ease.

We take pride in our accomplishments because our effort has manifested nearly everything that surrounds us. It has manifested our careers, our families, and our successes. That said, maybe something else—something bigger—has been with us the entire time, and when our actions match what is best for the greater good, everything falls into place. Maybe everything we have created and manifested in our life has arrived partly from our own doing and partly because there was a *letting go* involved. We did our best, we followed our heart, and then we let go of the outcome.

We create a more easeful, joyful existence when we enact some surrender around our pursuits. There is no need to worry about end results because we are held by the love of the Universe the entire time. Turn over your pain. Turn over your wondering. Know you have done what you can and let go.

PRACTICE 9
Walking through the Fire (Tapas)

Tapas is one of the five niyamas in the Eight Limbs of Yoga. Tapas refers to our discipline and also our restraint—not by renouncing all bad habits or trying to be perfect all the time but by adding a little discipline and appropriate restraint to our daily life, which goes a long way. In Sanskrit, *tapas* means "heat." We create physical heat during poses and asana. We create an emotional burn with continued meditation and introspection. Our practice, our discipline, becomes a fiery passion of showing up, doing our best, staying through flames and uncomfortable emotions, and then letting go. After any burn or discipline, there is new growth. By walking through the fire, we arrive a new person on the other side. What no longer serves us has been burned away, and we step into a new reality. With a little intentional, loving effort, we change.

DAY 241

Have you ever burned a letter, journal, or memento as a symbol of letting go? Have you ever written an old belief on a piece of paper, set it on fire, and watched it disappear? In high school, I used to burn love letters and all sorts of ridiculous objects as a symbol of an ended relationship. From the Sutras, "Tapas means 'to burn or create heat.' Anything burned out will be purified." The belief is that as the heat and flames disintegrate pages and words so, too, does the old thinking or behavior disappear. *Tapas* also translates to "self-discipline," and the practice of tapas reminds us of the purification that is possible out of pain or discomfort.[48]

Any discipline gets uncomfortable at times. A yoga and meditation practice is work and effort. Starting a new job or learning a new skill is difficult at first. Self-awareness, seeking, and introspection get really uncomfortable—maybe even "hot" or "burning."

Heat is a symptom of change. Fire is a symbol of growth. To get where we want to go, we might need to endure some heat and discomfort. We might need to let things burn. We might need to sit in the fire before we know what's waiting for us on the other side.

Get ready to turn up the heat. Get ready to focus on your disciplines, which lead to healing, growth, and change. If there's a goal you're trying to attain, now is the time. If there's a belief you're ready to let go, now is the time. If there's a letter or worry or emotion you want to burn, do it. For this practice, we're stepping into the fire.

....

48. Satchidananda, *The Yoga Sutras of Patanjali*, 75.

DAY 242
Sequoia Meditation

A few weeks after my husband moved out and it felt like my whole life was burning, I participated in a meditation series with Deepak Chopra and Oprah Winfrey. Chopra spoke of the thousand-year-old sequoia trees and how they germinate and spread. Apparently, it takes heat—a very hot fire—because only fire is hot enough to crack open the indestructible shells in order to spread the seeds. Chopra compared this to our human experience. Heat and burning isn't all bad. Forest fires kill a lot of vegetation, but they are necessary for others, including the sequoia, to thrive.[49] For me, Chopra's message was like a life vest. I grabbed onto the metaphor wholeheartedly; the image of the sequoia seeds gave me the comfort that maybe my tough exterior needed this current heat in order to crack open as well. Maybe this fiery place I was in wasn't doomsday like I thought. Maybe it was necessary for my growth.

If you are in a particularly challenging time or you feel like you are being consumed by emotions and discomfort you cannot handle, consider this lesson from the majestic sequoia. Is something being cracked open in you? Is it uncomfortable, and what other emotions arrive? For a moment, let yourself burn, and trust that discomfort is not always a sign that something is wrong. Some exteriors need fire in order to be opened and to promote growth.

....
49. Chopra 21-Day Meditation Experience.

DAY 243

When someone emerges from a situation better, stronger, and more capable, it is because they actually acknowledged themselves and their circumstance. Rather than run or hide, they allowed the difficult and painful sensations to arrive and burn. They sat in the fire and felt the swell of life rise inside them like hot coals. In doing so, they discovered new truth, which allowed them to pass through the fire and emerge a different version of themselves. The great thing is that you cannot do sitting in the fire wrong. (Unless you avoid it altogether.) You only need to be there for yourself, whatever that looks like in any given moment.

We are strong enough to sit in the fire despite our mind telling us we can't. We are capable of enduring great hardship and tragedy, and humans have proven this over and over again. Staying in the fire is not necessarily violent or sensational. Sometimes, acceptance of what is looks like taking a nap, meditating, or just doing absolutely nothing. Sometimes, strength, growth, and grace look oddly simple and unassuming. Like a seed that grows for the most part underground, unnoticed until its stem pushes through soil, most of our deep inner work happens underground too. Difficult experiences, whether on our mat or in life, must be acknowledged in order to transform us into something new. We are given the lesson and the insight only when we stay, patiently abiding, showing up, and not trying to bypass the process.

DAY 244

I believe there is something brilliant and magical about the times we feel defeated. Being humble and vulnerable enough to explore our grief can answer some really insightful questions, and it will then lead to healing—healing not only for the specific situation but from all situations where we have avoided the pain of being human. That's the cool thing about healing. As you expose and transform one pain point, you also heal others. Your reaction to any difficult situation is most likely a patterned reaction to any adversity, so every action and belief is a linked component and a clue to another. Knots that were formed years ago can be undone and released as the result of a present circumstance.

Recognizing our grief or pain—instead of locking it in the body, never looking or dealing with it again—helps it to move. Certain life experiences are sad, and we don't need to pretend otherwise. If you are sad, allow yourself to feel it. If you are angry, you don't need to push it away. Like our yoga practice has taught us, our role as the witness is to observe without judgment. Emotions that arrive will move, maybe quickly and maybe slowly, depending on the event. We honor ourselves when we look within and stay with what is there. As much as it is tempting to run to the next activity or distract yourself with food, substance, or relationships, take some time to sit down with yourself—not to analyze but simply to observe. Like interacting with a small child who is hurting, now is the time to listen to what needs care and attention. By offering yourself attention today, many old wounds could be healed as well.

DAY 245

We are fed many myths about yoga through images, media, and trends. As discussed in practice 2, yoga is more than a physical practice. There are seven other limbs beyond asana. Yoga is accessible to any body, shape, weight, or limitations. Yoga is not appearance, and it's not fashion. Yoga is a journey and a path to truth and enlightenment. Ancient yogis sought freedom from suffering through breath and meditation and by observing the mind. Physical postures were a way to observe discomfort and question pain.

If your physical practice is not how you want it to be, if you are being hard on your body and hard on yourself, consider the expectations you have and where they might come from. Is the image of yoga from society affecting your practice? Is the image of body from society affecting your practice? Remember that yoga is breath. Yoga is observing sensation. All of this can be done by a variety of different bodies, in a variety of different postures, and with infinite options and permission. Yoga helps us to be less concerned about how our body looks and more concerned about how our body feels. Surrender to the thoughts and criticisms that accompany your practice. Watch how the mind responds to discomfort or pain. Rather than hop out of the pain immediately or talk yourself out of a negative thought, can you instead lean in? Watch the pain shift, or watch your narrative around that pain shift. We stay in our practice not with a forceful willfulness but gently and with the sole intention of honoring where we are.

DAY 246

After some time spent engaged in any discipline, whether it's a yoga practice, a daily meditation, a new exercise routine, a hobby, a project, or even parenthood and relationships, we start to feel the burn of tapas. If we are engaged in tapas, we might feel discomfort, doubt, or like giving up. There is a difference between fear and the fire. Burning is a result of staying with our uncomfortable emotions or experience. Fear is running away, avoiding, or being in denial.

It's important to know when fear is trying to pull us away from our discipline. The mind will say we can't. The mind will ask, "*Who are you to do this?*" The mind will create a million distractions and excuses. Tapas is a wonderful opportunity to recognize the difference between our mind and our intuition. Notice the thoughts that attempt to derail you from your practice, and ask yourself compassionately, "*What is true and real?*" Just because something feels uncomfortable does not mean we need to leave or change it. Like during a yoga pose that requires our strength and effort, some discomfort is okay and even necessary in order to change and grow.

As we let go, as we burn past beliefs and behaviors, as we keep moving forward through the fire, there is bound to be discomfort and new sensations. Observe the new with clear eyes and nonjudgment. New can feel intimidating but not because you are incapable or unworthy. Just like muscles that have not been used will feel tired or sore, behaviors that are new in your life will feel foreign before they shift to feeling natural. Fear will tell you to get out, but what happens when you stay?

DAY 247

If you can ride out the discomfort, you will find a new strength and even a new Self on the other side. Remember that yoga teaches us to welcome in all sensations—good, bad, easy, joyful, and uncomfortable. We try not to name them, although our mind desperately wants to label. Dig deep into your intuition and your body, and trust that you are allowed a full experience. The same way we can make the choice to return to the breath or stay in a pose, we can also make the choice to remain in the fires and trials of life. Staying does not look like forcing, overdoing, or unnecessarily pushing. Staying does not look like yelling or criticizing yourself. We can grant ourselves the grace and the mercy that exist within any period of change. If you're experiencing the fire, if you're engaged in tapas, be kind. Kindness through change might take reassessing our beliefs about how we achieve goals.

As James Kingsland writes, "*Facing down* is typically how we do things in the West. With mindfulness, we actually teach people to become curious."[50] Curiosity takes the force out of staying. Rather than push ourselves, we calmly abide in order to learn something new. We approach all sensations as equal, not labeling any as appropriate, good, or bad. A "good" meditation or yoga practice is one where we observed, and it's not necessarily a practice that felt comfortable all the time. By removing the belief that progress requires pushing, we take better care of ourselves and can stay with difficult emotions through a lens of compassion and true awareness.

....
50. Kingsland, *Siddhārtha's Brain*, 156.

DAY 248

Every yogi questions their own practice at times. No matter how long anyone has been practicing, there is always more to learn and more mistakes to learn from. Yoga is not about finding "the answer" and then having nothing to do or work on after that. So, if you are still seeking, still practicing, still making mistakes, but with awareness, then you are doing the practice right.

Be careful if you use your yoga practice as another way to treat yourself poorly or self-criticize. We embark on our practice with utmost understanding that our seeking and our curiosity often leads to more questions. Our trial and error leads to more clarity. Our witnessing leads to more enlightenment.

To practice tapas, we must feel the burn of the fire and stay open to the lessons within the discomfort. We don't expect that anything worthwhile will not cause some pain. We treat ourselves with compassion and kindness along the way. We can even ask ourselves if difficult emotions are bad or if anything needs labeling at all. Of course we feel sad when something ends. Of course we feel scared when something new begins. Of course we feel joy with accomplishment. Your emotions are not the enemy. Stay. Witness. Feel. Allow emotions to come and pass through. Maybe you can feel an emotion without the need to react. The emotion itself never causes harm, but our reactions and attachments can be violent or cause more pain. Not only are all emotions temporary, but they require no reaction at all.

DAY 249

What is a discipline? Does it have a negative association in our society? Personally, when I think of a discipline, words such as *hard*, *stern*, *forced*, *strict*, and *serious* come to mind. Maybe you can think of others. Language is very affected by culture, so concepts and words take on subtle meanings and associations based on that society and time period. In yoga, our discipline is probably much softer than the idea we have in our mind. Our discipline is compassionate, loving, forgiving, and kind. Our discipline is our practice and how we show up for ourselves.

Unlike we may have been taught, engaging in a discipline does not mean we show up to prove a point or because we feel forced. We show up because we love ourselves and are seeking. We show up because we are humble and don't know where else to go. We show up because we have faith that our yoga will bring us something we need. We show up as we are, right now, with nothing to hide. Our discipline explores our intentions and our truthfulness. Our discipline is an opportunity to practice our beliefs on the mat.

So, really, *tapas* translated to "discipline" may not feel good at first and may not even be accurate. Depending on our experience, the word *discipline* might bring up harsh images that make you feel unmotivated, even scared. Discipline in yoga is not a punishment. Through the discipline of our practice, we learn how to take care of ourselves and treat ourselves with more kindness. The fruits of our discipline reveal the power of showing up in love rather than harshness.

DAY 250
Matsyasana (Supported Fish Pose)

Grab a blanket or towel and roll it up so it can be placed longways across your mat, parallel to the short edge. Place the blanket under your shoulder blades and lie down on your back. Position yourself so your arms rest above the blanket, outstretched and away from your body, like a T. Be sure the back of your head is able to rest on the ground. This is matsyasana, a heart opener. You do not need much height from the blanket or towel, so make the roll shorter if you need to. You should be able to lie comfortably, without strain in the low back. Do this for five to ten minutes at a time, in the morning or before bed. Close your eyes and breathe.

Matsyasana opens the heart and stretches the muscles and ligaments across the front of your chest and under your arms. As I lie and breathe in this pose, I observe moments of resistance, possibly from my heart being open and exposed. I feel a bit vulnerable, and staying in the pose is not always comfortable from an emotional standpoint. My body and my cells somewhat cringe at baring my heart to the sky, at pulling on the muscles that are used to drawing inward and expanding my chest with each telling inhale. Staying in the fire means knowing when a pose is too much or when we can observe despite discomfort or a desire to move. Even though matsyasana elicits a nervous response from my body, part of me knows that the pose is necessary and beneficial. Often, the pose we resist is the one we need.

DAY 251

Just like we have the choice to come out of a pose when it is too much for the body, we also have a choice in how we practice mindfulness during challenging times. If you are dealing with grief, trauma, loss, depression, or anxiety, there is no need to push yourself beyond what your emotions can handle right now. The concept of tapas invites us to embrace our full experience as long as we are not causing more harm than healing. As always, you get to decide when you can stay and when you need to bow out. Yoga is a powerful practice. Postures and breath move energy and unearth emotions. We need to be able to discern when we are ready and able to experience certain pain points. I had a student who did not like cat/cow. It turns out her resistance to the pose was more than dislike. The movement brought up memories of a childhood trauma, so we found ways to modify. Seated cat/cow was a more pleasant experience for her. There are always ways to adapt your practice, and these acts of self-care provide much healing. No one ever has the right to force you into doing a posture or to push you beyond your level of comfort. When trauma survivors are able to practice choice and advocate for themselves, they recover pieces of identity that had been lost to their perpetrators. Practicing tapas is not intended to push you into further suffering. There is no rush on your healing path, and adapting your practice out of compassion and awareness is a beautiful way to take care of yourself, especially during difficult times.

DAY 252

It's very common to hear people at twelve-step meetings talk about how their guilt and shame over being an alcoholic led to even more damaging drinking. For an alcoholic, waking up after a binge produces so much guilt that they often feel they have no way to calm the self-loathing mind except by taking another drink. And so, on the cycle repeats. Tapas helps us acknowledge a pattern long enough to understand what is happening. With awareness, we can make a small change. To break a pattern, Stephen Cope suggests "to interrupt [the pattern] just at its very endpoint."[51]

Just at its endpoint ... I think of this as the beautiful and crucial space that exists right before we give in to a pattern—the space where we have a choice. It might be painful to pause and observe ourselves rather than react, but by restraining from acting, we gain truth into our behavior. We usually know what our unattractive or unhealthy habits are. We know if we tell small lies or never show up on time. We know if we run to food or substance or shopping to ease feelings of inadequacy. The discipline of tapas asks us to pause before reaction. Eating one slice of cake does not mean we might as well eat the whole thing. We can stop our guilt and self-loathing in its tracks by choosing a new pattern, by practicing a little restraint, and noticing how we feel when we do. How do we feel when we stop eating at half the cake? We have just interrupted an unhealthy behavior. Instead of deepening the groove, of feeding the samskara, we have made room for a new way.

....
51. Cope, *The Wisdom of Yoga*, 154.

DAY 253

I started spontaneously crying in the car. Everything was fine, and all of a sudden, I felt the tightness in my chest and the welling up behind my eyes. The tears came. I probably went entire years without crying. It didn't matter if I wanted to cry because I was happy or because I was sad. I simply didn't let my body allow it. I changed the subject, changed the radio station, or changed my location. I ran. I numbed. I critiqued.

We are conditioned to figure everything out. We think every emotion needs a reason or a justification. *Is this big enough for a good cry?* Sometimes, the body simply needs release. I am reminded of my dog who instinctively stops in the middle of anything and shakes from head to tail. The energy let out and released is palpable throughout the room and around her form. She emerges from the experience a different dog. The dog doesn't worry or consider why. The dog doesn't feel guilty when it's done. She moves on as if it never happened.

Energy wants to move. Energy will arrive as sensation—a thirst, a hunger, a need to rest, or a need to cry. Not everything needs a label or an answer. Not everything needs figuring out. Our role when we feel something in the body approaching is to allow it.

Let yourself dance. Let yourself scream. Let yourself cry. Spontaneous release means letting go of the conditioned desire to keep it all together and to maintain a pretty outer appearance. Sometimes, release is exactly what the body (and the soul) needs.

DAY 254

What happens when you don't get the job you really want? How do you talk to yourself after you read the rejection letter? Do phrases like *I interview terribly*, *I never should have tried to get that job in the first place*, and *Who do I think I am?* float to the surface of your mind? Worse, do you actually internalize and believe those words? Maybe you believe the words so much you start to sell yourself short, so you apply for a job that is beneath you. You ensure success by playing life small and avoiding the burn.

Tapas helps us practice becoming aware of the critical voice and refraining from internalizing it. We don't need to pile self-criticism onto an already hurtful situation. Feeding the voice loses us in story and prevents us from staying with our true experience. I used to think something was drastically wrong with my self-esteem and my psyche because I had such a continual stream of negative thoughts in my head. I wondered about all the ways internalizing my experiences had affected my choices.

Tapas helps us acknowledge our hurt while becoming aware of the critical voice. When something bad happens, like when we don't get the job we really want, our partner rejects us, or we make a mistake, we don't need to beat ourselves up. We don't need to buy into the story that the experience has anything to do with *who we are* at our core. Everyone gets rejected. Everyone screws up—sometimes big and sometimes small. Practice softening your inner critic when life doesn't go your way or you get hurt. Acknowledge your hurt more than the lying voice in your head.

DAY 255

Tapas is a wonderful practice in teaching us the benefits of pain. First, painful experiences alert us that a change might need to be made. Second, pain purifies emotional knots and heals wounds from the past; it also grants wisdom on the other side. Still, who likes pain? This quote from the Sutras makes me question my relationship to pain: "We will actually be happy to receive pain if we keep in mind its purifying effects."[52] How lovely, but really?! Can you imagine thanking someone who caused you pain? The lesson here is not so unattainable. It is probably a stretch to thank the person for causing us pain—at least at first. However, we can practice tapas in our relationships by learning from our reaction, especially when someone hurts us. Maybe you have reacted to someone causing you pain by ignoring them, yelling at them, or some other retaliatory response. I used to retaliate. When my partner hurt me, for example, I lashed out at him, called him names, and in general tried to get back at his words or actions. Sometimes, I behaved rudely toward others, letting my pain ripple out to innocent bystanders. Interestingly, this sort of reaction never made me feel better. I still felt hurt and pain.

When you are hurt, practice the restraint of tapas. Rather than retaliate, which always made me feel worse, treat yourself with more kindness. We don't need to return pain to others just because we are in pain. The person who really needs love and kindness is you.

....
52. Satchidananda, *The Yoga Sutras of Patanjali*, 75.

DAY 256

Recently I considered how much my yoga practice has shifted and changed over years and life circumstances. When newly sober and newly single, I craved a fiery practice that allowed me to burn through anger and regret while strengthening my muscles and sense of self. A few years later, I gravitated toward slow, gentle (and nearly still) movements that provided deep introspection. On day 46 I talk about hovering in phalakasana (plank pose) and how it allowed tears and difficult emotions to emerge. In plank, I felt permission to cry.

For you, it might be plank pose that gets you through a difficult time. It may also be child's pose, goddess, or staying still for a few minutes in shavasana. Whatever your style or the pose your body currently craves, a regular practice will bring deep insight into what goes on in your mind when you're up against a wall. Do you lie down and give up? Do you blame or yell at yourself? Or do you find out what you're capable of?

Yoga is a practice that honors the comeback. We fall apart in order to put ourselves back together. If you're weak, yoga will make you strong. If you're confused, yoga will bring you clarity. If you're lost, yoga will lead you to self-discovery. These are my beliefs. Take a few minutes a day, morning or night, to practice your pose; see how quickly the pose progresses, as does your self-confidence. One day at a time, you'll hold the pose longer. That's the power of practice.

DAY 257

You don't have to be an addict to embrace a life of presence without numbing. Your most authentic life comes from accepting all your emotions and desires. There will always be a substance or patterned reaction of some kind to pull us away from ourselves. Just like a drug addict learns to observe sensation without getting out the needle, we can observe ourselves the moment before we decide to react—the moment before we decide to smoke, eat, not eat, throw up, shop, lie, or gossip. Each moment we make a different choice, we change our brain's reaction to life.

I was given a lot of strategies to handle alcohol cravings. If you go to a party, bring nonalcoholic options. When a craving arrives, call a supportive friend or your sponsor. If the craving feels really overwhelming, go for a run or drop and start doing push-ups. Cravings for alcohol were like fires on my skin. I had to notice, wait, and watch them pass. Researchers have found mindfulness to be an effective tool to help overcome any addiction.[53] For the addict, cravings are a tiny, tremendous moment of truth. Illuminating this tiny moment can prevent relapse. Yoga teaches us to notice sensations, which means acknowledging the burn of desire and observing it without reaction. Don't reach for the substance. Don't repeat the normal pattern. Stay in the fire of observing, and when you don't reach for the drug of choice, you have not only overcome the craving but also shifted your brain's reaction to being in the fire.

....

53. Kingsland, *Siddārtha's Brain*, 161.

DAY 258

Decision paralysis. The rumination. The obsession. The inability to do anything until we know what is *right* and what is *wrong*. Feelings of unease may point to something needing to be let go, but it's not always what we think. Instead of remaining paralyzed or making a quick decision out of panic, move forward slowly, and make small decisions that will reveal more along your path. First, I decided to go to yoga. Then, I found a therapist. I tried church. I prioritized more self-care and more time with my kids. I met friends for coffee and searched for different careers. During any decision-making process, we can move forward in small ways until the path becomes clearer.

If there is a decision to be made, open yourself up to feelings and signs, and move forward with all possibilities instead of clinging to one result that you believe will solve all your problems. Harsh decisions might be necessary, but they often are not the full story. Feeling bored in your job or neglected in your relationship doesn't mean either need to end. There are other options, such as talking to someone or doing some inner work. You don't need to wait until you know exactly what to do. Tiny decisions along the way will guide and point you to the perfect ending, which may not be what you expected. You won't make the *wrong* decision because you will be collecting more information along the way. One small healthy choice a day moves you forward on your intended path and gently reveals more as you go. Meaningful change is slow and steady; it is a continued discipline, not a magic bullet.

DAY 259

"Yoga found me." I have heard many people say this about how they came to practice yoga. I don't disagree. I started practicing yoga with my mom when I was fifteen, having no idea that the practice would see me through some of my most difficult times. The discipline of tapas prepares us for the inevitable challenges and tragedies of life. We practice on the days we feel good so we are wiser, stronger, and more faithful on the days we feel bad. Tapas creates our depth and builds our character so that we can remain present for our full experience, whether that experience is painful, heart-wrenching, or joyous. Many people walk into a yoga class at some sort of low point. They seek peace, healing, answers, or strength. Yoga fulfills its promise by inviting us to turn inward, to dig deep and muster the courage to admit how we feel, to take an honest look, and to burn—if necessary. Yes, it is the difficult moments that bring us to our knees and teach us of our capacity to rise. It is the tragedies and hardships that shape us and teach us the most about who we are and what we can endure. As we return to our daily discipline, as we show up on our mat and in our relationships, we build character that will see us through times of desperation. When we allow ourselves to burn— rather than moving through an experience in denial—we learn something new about ourselves or the world. We don't leave residue of an experience behind because we acknowledge our emotions in the present. After, we are pure and free.

DAY 260

Tapas invites us to do one small thing and to be consistent. Often, we try to fix everything at once; life gets out of hand, and we want to change everything too quickly. How can we tighten our gaze in order to stay with what is right now? Instead of piling on a monstrous undertaking and then abandoning ship when you can't follow through, choose an attainable, close-up goal. Choose a honed-in view. Choose something you can maintain and show up for. My yoga practice started small. I showed up with my mat, and I breathed. That was my only undertaking—to breathe for the entire hour.

Doing one small thing *can* change your life. The greatest part is: you don't have to know where the new thing will lead you. Looking back, yoga and meditation strengthened my intuition and my ability to trust myself. So, a few years later when I really needed these qualities, I had them. Lately, my one small thing has been drinking a glass of water upon waking, before I have my coffee. This small act has already accomplished a few things. First, I start my day with an intention of health and cleansing. Second, I notice the mornings I don't feel like drinking the water—why do I resist something quite easy and good for me?

What is one small thing you can do for now? Do you need to eliminate something? Do you need to add a glass of water? Do you need to try an earlier bedtime or a walk in the afternoon? Watch in wonderment as your one small thing creates larger ripples and, eventually, entire shifts in course you hadn't even considered.

DAY 261

There's a term in recovery rooms called the *pink cloud*. It's the period of exhilaration when you glimpse your life free from the drug. People float into meetings on a high, a few weeks or months sober, all of a sudden with an expanded view of life. They see life without addiction, life without a crutch. They catch air and view what it might be like to live this way forever. No more hangovers. No more numbing and running. Just facing and owning their emotions. From rock bottom to endless possibility, people taste freedom.

Now that they've done this thing—the thing they never thought possible—they start to wonder, *"What else can I do that I didn't see?"*

Embarking on a quest brings tail-wagging excitement upon anticipation. But in the middle of the process, as the new way of life gets uncomfortable, difficult, even aching, your mind forgets the initial euphoria, and you wonder if all of it was a dream or, worse, a crazy, futile aspiration. Eventually, the pink cloud wears off, and you settle into the effort of getting healthy, showing up to a discipline, or removing a damaging behavior. You battle through sore muscles that are learning new strength, and you face the relentless, critical voice that says you think you can do this but you can't and that none of it even matters. I think it's important to revisit the cloud, to remember why we are here, and to remind ourselves that just because our effort is difficult does not mean it's not worthwhile. Choosing to stay with the discipline is when our effort really pays off. The pink cloud got us over the initial hump, and now, the meaningful work begins.

DAY 262

When I stand on one leg in tree pose, the test is always to turn my head to one side and look out across the opposite shoulder of my lifted leg. Almost always, I *fall*. What seemed so strong and grounded while looking ahead becomes extremely wobbly once I adjust my view. The exercise reminds me there is always another point of growth. There is always another way to experience the same posture. Sometimes, our practice becomes boring and too easy. We have reached another edge and are asked yet again, *"Are you still willing?"* We can acknowledge where we have progressed and where there is still room to grow. For every obstacle we overcome, there is more to remind us of our discipline. I love that the same yoga pose can continue to be a teacher even after years of practice. Common poses, such as tree or downward-facing dog, provide infinite opportunities to explore and grow. *What happens when I engage my core like this? What if I press more firmly into my standing foot? What if I lengthen through the crown of my head? What shifts? Where have I gained new awareness and insight?*

Sometimes, physical setbacks are the best ways to explore new views. We may be accustomed to always doing cat/cow pose on our knees but, for whatever reason, this option becomes unavailable, so we must find a new way. Cat/cow can be done seated or standing. We might have never had the chance to explore this new way had we not been limited and basically forced. Welcome any opportunity to try something different. Meet every edge with grace and willingness. Your growth will be never ending.

DAY 263

To get from *here* to *there*, we must put in consistent effort, and the small pieces add up over time. We mistakenly believe that big dreams and big goals must take tremendous force or dramatic effort to attain. We are impatient and want to see results now. But actually, consistent practice is what creates lifelong, sustainable change. Each day has twenty-four hours. Meditating for ten minutes each day eventually creates a whole new person. Writing one page a day is how you produce a thick manuscript. Holding balance postures, even while falling in and out, produces a strong core. You are better off practicing yoga for twenty minutes a day than attending an hour-and-a-half class once a month. Short, consistent effort pays off more than crash diets or extreme measures.

Beyond the physical postures, yoga is a lifestyle. During a traffic jam or a hard day, we have our breath. Before an important meeting or conversation, we know how to close our eyes and ask our heart for advice. When someone wrongs us, we learn to acknowledge their experience as well as our own. Yoga lives inside us and supports us because we practice every day, not necessarily on the mat each time but in the way we treat the body, talk to ourselves and others, and make choices. Pretty soon, all our yoga stacks up, and we realize we are not the same person as we were when we started. People may even start to notice the change in you and ask what you are doing differently. They want the answer to an easeful life. There is no easy fix; it's the daily yoga practice, which has now become part of who you are.

DAY 264

There are stories of yogis engaging in extreme practices, such as depriving themselves or putting their bodies through harsh elements, in order to experience the purifying effects of pain. While we don't need to torture the body, we can learn something from enduring a little discomfort about staying, acceptance, and the workings of the mind. According to the Sutras, "The power to control the body and senses comes by *tapasya*. If we accept everything, what can affect us?"[54]

My family plunges into frigid Lake Superior every November for a brief moment of ice cold on our skin. The hardest part for me is the ten minutes or so before jumping in, anticipating the cold, wondering about the sensation, and wanting to stay warm by the fire. As it turns out, the lead-up is always more daunting than the actual event. We jump in and out so quickly, and of course it's cold, but there's an element of accomplishment once finished. Plus, the body feels quite refreshed. While we certainly don't need to starve ourselves or risk self-harm, we can learn from experiences that push the body into a bit of discomfort. We can watch the mind and what it says, observing that our stories are often worse than the reality. Whether you stay for a few extra breaths in a challenging pose or dive into a lake on a cold day, practices that contradict the mind and awaken our senses help us to accept other discomforts in life and, as a bonus, bring a smile at the end of our accomplishment.

....
54. Satchidananda, *The Yoga Sutras of Patanjali*, 139.

DAY 265

It is a bold claim to think that life will not affect us, that we will not be hurt by someone's words or actions, that we will not be shattered by the reality of loss or enduring. Yoga does not promise to take away our pain or our troubles. Yoga offers wisdom in meeting life where it is, especially that which is out of our control. Acceptance means much more than taking an apathetic viewpoint or not caring when something is hurtful or unfair. A difficult but powerful question we can ask ourselves when going through any amount of difficulty is *"Can I allow this experience to become part of my journey?"* We are forever shaped by our experiences and our handling of them. Is it possible that a cancer diagnosis can lead us on a path to acceptance? Is it possible to forgive someone who has betrayed us? Can we lean into our pain rather than turn away? Yoga teaches us that turning toward our discomfort is the path to an awakened life. This is not about finding the "silver lining" or the reason why. Acceptance is about acknowledging all the injustices and uncertainties and leaning in anyway, feeling all the tough emotions.

Something could be clearing out. Something could be making space for new growth. We do not determine what we are given in order to shape us along our path. Lessons are chosen for us through experiences we may not have wished for. Blessings are revealed but only when we keep moving forward. We do not have to go as far as being grateful for our pain, although with time, this can happen too. For now, it is enough to stay.

DAY 266

There may be a part of you wondering if you have the strength to keep going, wondering if all of these practices are worth it. I am referring to your yoga practice or anything else happening in your life. Consider ways that you can show up gently rather than forcing or yelling. Understand that disciplines get challenging. What is your reaction? How do you behave when the fire gets hot? At any edge in life, we feel the pull to turn back. We wonder if the safety and familiarity of the past is better than the unknown. The edge is a turning point. Yes, you can always go back, or you can muster the courage to continue forward despite fear, despite doubt. Our wounds and our demons will present immediately before new insight is reached.

My teacher had us in goddess pose, a wide-legged squat. We had been there for several minutes, and I was looking forward to standing up. My thighs quivered and shook. I pressed my palms together more firmly and tried to hold on. She said we would stay there for five more minutes—five excruciating minutes! Of course, we had the option to stand up anytime. *But could we stay?* Curious, I stayed. I figured I wouldn't die. I noticed my anxiousness and self-doubt and wondered at how little I thought of my own strength. When it was time, I slowly straightened my legs and rose out of the pose. I thought I might fall over as my legs went to jelly as if giving up. I made it. For days after, I confidently walked through my life, recalling that moment and remembering that I am stronger than I think.

DAY 267

A translation of *tapas* that I love is "uplifting discipline." Again, we do not need to interpret discipline as something harsh or punishing. Any discipline requires some level of restraint and commitment, but the intention is to approach any effort with a quality of friendliness, kindness, and joy. Think of tapas as eating a delicious but healthy meal. Even though you are forgoing the pleasure of something sweet, the experience can be just as enjoyable, especially when you consider the health benefits to your body. Tackling a project can be met with joy and inspiration, knowing the end result will produce something new and rewarding. Walking every day will bring more energy and aliveness. Eating healthy will increase your well-being and change your physique. All of these daily disciplines lead to beautiful outcomes.

Our attitude has a lot to do with the success of our effort. If we arrive to our mat chastising our body or critical of the poses we can't do, not only will the process feel terrible along the way but the outcome will be affected. A critical voice is never helpful to our efforts. If your goal is to stay longer in boat pose, approach this posture with love rather than force. Keep your feet down, or use your hands on your knees for support. Your core is still getting stronger. Your body is still changing. One day, you will be able to float your feet off the mat and extend your arms. How are you affecting your practice with criticism rather than kindness? Disciplines focused on healthy outcomes are meant to be enjoyed. Don't miss the gift of the process.

DAY 268

I forgot to meet someone for coffee. We arranged the appointment days before, but I didn't write it down, and I never showed up. An hour or so after we were supposed to meet, he texted me with a smiley face. "I guess I'll allow one no-show."

I felt terrible. Immediately my body erupted into anxiety and guilt. I backtracked in my mind and tried to figure out where I went wrong. I began writing him back that my kids were the reason, that I hadn't put in my calendar, that I was tired … Then, I deleted everything and simply wrote, "I'm sorry. I forgot."

We are allowed to make mistakes—even though it brings up uncomfortable emotions. I don't know why I feel the need to constantly present myself as perfect. I would certainly forgive a friend for not showing up or forgetting something. Why can't I lend myself the same compassion? Not allowing ourselves to make mistakes or not being able to give a genuine apology keeps us separate; the ego remains strong, and we lose our connection to our true Self. No one benefits when we try to hide our imperfections behind excuses or justifications. We are not above or different from others. Like everyone, we are capable of error. As tapas teaches us, staying with our discomfort is when change and growth happen. Even though it may feel more comfortable to have a great excuse for missing an appointment or showing up late, an honest, genuine apology helps both people to feel better. A genuine apology removes judgment and superiority, and it helps everyone to move forward because we all can recognize our humanness.

DAY 269

It's hard to see the falls and setbacks as blessings when you're in the middle of picking yourself up. If you're at the beginning and it's that horrendous, pride-sucking, ego-dissolving time to drag yourself back, let me remind you that nothing is lost. Our egos get quite angry when they are being questioned, weakened, and chiseled away to reveal our connection to the Divine. Your ego will fight back with shame, blame, and fear. Because of your ego, you will want to crawl into a dark hole and never come out. You will want to wallow in all the ways you can't seem to get it right. You will call yourself worthless and hopeless. This is your ego fighting for first place in your mind.

The comeback is a great opportunity to deflate the ego and step into your own truth. Yes, you screwed up. Yes, you tried again and failed. It's okay. There is no need to get everything right the first few times. The only way to avoid falling is to never take the leap. The only way to avoid humility is to never step into something new. When I look back on all my falls and setbacks, I realize that's when I witnessed grace. Grace entered when I felt I had nothing and no one left, not even myself. Getting back up is worth it. Getting back up takes guts, and it is damn beautiful. Your getting back up will inspire others. No one needs to hear a story about a perfect path. Learn from your mistakes, hold your head high with grace and humanness, and keep going.

DAY 270

We are not defined by the one final outcome to which we assign a label but more by all the tiny decisions we made along the way, all the ways we honored our experience and didn't run, all on our search for Self. *Married, divorced, parent, childless, single, sober, employed, writer, yogi*… The label never does justice to the journey. Sometimes, writing feels like typing one letter, one word, or one excruciating sentence at a time. Sometimes, yoga feels like plunking heavy and unwilling limbs into postures. Sometimes, true love feels like stepping back, accepting yourself, and watching a gentle snow fall rather than focusing on another person. Labels give the illusion of perfect paths as well as a box for our identity. But the true Self is a culmination of experience, how we reacted, and what we did to handle emotions along the way. The Self is cultivated through energy and allowing; we can allow for an experience or resist it. We can move gracefully through or kick and scream in retaliation.

If you have arrived at your perfect ending, enjoy the moment, as it will change. If you are battling a hardship, trust that acceptance is the path to overcoming. During challenging times, we can engage in behaviors that make us feel grounded, such as practicing yoga, fostering healthy relationships, and resting, or we can dismiss our experience with numbing behaviors, such as substance abuse, overspending, or any other immediate gratification that pulls us away from our experience. If we are tempted to reach for something else, tapas asks us to stay. So, when the experience passes, as it will, we arrive at the new destination centered, grateful, and able to see how we have grown.

DAY 271

When we feel pain, we want to get as far away from it as possible. I have literally tried to outrun pain by getting in the car or tying up my running shoes. I have tried to drown pain with alcohol and suffocate pain by starving myself. I have written my pain down, torn it into tiny pieces, and set it ablaze. Sometimes, my avoidance is not so dramatic; I simply dismiss that I am in any pain at all and move it to the bottom of my to-do list.

Despite all my efforts to shuffle my pain to the bottom of the heap, it resurfaces. Like a thousand little stones that keep washing up on shore, my pain may get swept into the ocean for a bit, but the tide of a new day or a new experience always brings it back to me.

Reluctantly, I pick up my pain. I hold it in my hand and feel its weight. I turn it over in my palm and resist every urge I have to throw it back. After a while of walking with my pain, I notice it is not so heavy. I even find some gratitude and tenderness for the burden. Now, I am on the lookout, attempting to find the ugliest, scraggliest piece of hurt from my past so I can wipe it off and hold it in my heart like a secret treasure. I no longer want to throw it all back. I no longer want to ignore my experience or myself. I want to be free. By looking at all my pain at once, carrying it with me and watching it get lighter from exposure, I've realized pain doesn't feel so scary anymore.

PRACTICE 10
Truth (Satya)

What is true? What is real? These two essential and profound questions I learned from Kripalu can be asked regarding every thought, every situation, and every life event for which we seek clarity and understanding. By asking yourself these questions, you acknowledge the power of perception and the willingness to explore a more open, compassionate view. *Satya* is one of the five yamas of Patanjali's Yoga Sutras, and it means "truth."[55] From a place of truth, we behave with integrity, honoring the moment instead of an expectation. The truth is not always pleasant, but it is real. To practice satya, we no longer lie to ourselves or others. We no longer hide behind façades that build resentment. We no longer fear our dark parts because when illuminated, they may be addressed. The truth is always beneficial for our own healing and for our contentment. Satya allows us to be present with what is, and in practicing this beautiful tenet, we meet life with more ease and less resistance.

....
55. Satchidananda, *The Yoga Sutras of Patanjali*, 118.

DAY 272

Existing beneath the lens of needing to be someone is exhausting. If I am at a party or an event, I almost instinctively try to discern who someone wants me to be, and I attempt to fit that. What does that person look like? How do they act, and what do they believe? I can sense when I am betraying myself, and it feels very superficial to try and get everyone's approval. Satya teaches us to live from the inside-out rather than the outside-in. A lot of our unhappiness comes when we resist something from within that wants to come out or when we act in a way that goes against ourselves. We try to fit into an acceptable version instead of allowing ourselves to be unique. We silence our voice or our opinion out of fear of what someone will think. This maintenance in order to be likable is not only dishonest but unsustainable. We all hold multiple roles and identities, but at the center, there is always us. Whether I am in a group of mothers, writers, yogis, or wives, I can express myself in a way that includes all of these parts of me as well as the parts that may be unexpected or even contradictory. Your truth is yours and doesn't need to fit into a form. Sure, there may be consequences to voicing our truth—everyone may not like us—but it is much better to like ourselves, to honor our truth, and to let the Universe handle the rest instead of constantly manipulating a situation that will never produce real meaning or genuine connection.

DAY 273

Satya is at the heart of any mindfulness practice because it encourages an open view of our moment-to-moment experience and the nature of reality. Buddhist teachings encourage an "observational quality of attention" as well as compassion for our experience in order to reach pure awareness.[56] Reality is full of emotions and sensations, pleasant and unpleasant. To become aware of our shifting experience is to meet the truth of our existence.

From this standpoint, the technique of our practice is not as important as our acceptance and awareness of what is. Just because you are able to do a posture, for example, doesn't mean it is appropriate for you in any given moment. What worked during your practice yesterday may not be the same today. When we remain open, we are always seeking and investigating our experience. We never reach a point of "getting it" because we understand the impermanent nature of reality. You might have a morning routine or a way of moving through postures. But if a posture doesn't "feel" right in the moment, choose something else. There are times during a yoga class when I am able to watch my ego and discern what my body actually needs. The instructor offers a posture, and while I know I am physically able to complete it, I choose to rest in child's pose. As you remain open and observing, you will notice when your ego is pushing you and when your body is speaking to you through sensation or subtle energy. Always honor the body where it is. This is a powerful practice in truth and mindfulness.

....
56. Treleaven, *Trauma-Sensitive Mindfulness*, 60–61.

DAY 274

There are not a lot of places in life where you can tell it like it is. I tell small lies to my doctors, therapists, children, colleagues, family, and friends. "Yes, I floss every day." "I'm late because there was traffic." "No, nothing is bothering me." I've learned to love and appreciate the places I can voice my truth and have it respected. Recovery groups are a great example. We share vulnerabilities and ugly truths without the risk of judgment. Likewise, we know people will call us out if we are misguided or missing something. Sometimes, we need our blind spots to be pointed out, and when someone is brave enough to do this for us, it feels very nurturing, not mean. Telling someone what they want to hear produces no deep thoughts or curiosity and, therefore, no road to change.

This doesn't mean we get to go around telling everyone what we think is wrong with them. Satya is not an excuse to judge or attack others. But if someone is actively seeking help and asking your advice, giving them some kindly worded truth can be the most loving thing to do. Safe people and spaces that can hear your truth without judgment offer a great amount of support in the form of listening and connection. Our most intimate relationships are formed when we feel permission to say something we are afraid to admit. Choose your safe people wisely. You don't need to be chastised or berated as a result of being vulnerable. Likewise, if someone is being vulnerable with you, consider how a little honesty, gently delivered, can be the best way to love them.

DAY 275

Debbie Ford calls the masks we wear "shells of protection" and says, "There is great value in understanding what we hide behind."[57] When I read her words, I am reminded of the soft turtle safe inside a tough exterior or the fragile snail that needs its shell to move and survive. Very young, we learn what elicits approval and what our parents or caregivers expect from us. As we get older, we apply this learned skill to more things in life. We adopt roles, we create masks to hide shameful emotions, and we don layers of protection to shield us from pain. We attach our identity to someone else's smile instead of our own heart. We attach our worth to someone else's words, a paycheck, or a new title instead of relying on our own sense of Self.

We believe in the roles so intently that we forget we are wearing masks in the first place. Our masks become our personality. Humor covers sadness. Shyness covers hurt. Achievement covers inadequacy. Admitting our soft center takes awareness of the whole Self. Any masks we wear have great purpose and were necessary for our survival. Not being aware of the mask and what it's protecting prevents us from ever removing it once the mask no longer serves us, once the shell becomes detrimental to who we are today. You can take off the mask whenever and with whomever you choose. You can use the mask as a teacher and a way into your true Self. We have the power to compassionately look within and remove the masks with an awareness of our whole Self in order to exist and share as our most authentic version today.

....
57. Ford, *The Dark Side of the Light Chasers*, 55.

DAY 276

There are no rules about how your life needs to look. The family, the relationship, the job, the pursuits—none of them need to match a societal norm. Often, we get attached to the promise, the promise of an ideal family, a two-car garage, or whatever image we have in our head about what will make us happy. We stay tied to a narrow idea and spend our time trying to fit in instead of seeing other more creative solutions that may be better for our circumstance.

When I got divorced, my ex-husband and I were required by the state of Wisconsin to take a coparenting class. I was annoyed, but the class turned out to be extremely informative. I thought we might be lectured, but the facilitator delivered a much more compassionate view of family after divorce. She explained that our new family didn't need to match married couples or even what other separated parents do. As long as we kept the best interest of the children in mind, our holidays, schedules, and day-to-day could look like anything we wanted. Being divorced did not mean we no longer had love or a stable family; it just looked different now. Whatever your situation, return to the essential question of *"What is true?"* Does a loving family need two parents under the same roof? What makes a stable, healthy childhood? Can a committed relationship look different from marriage? Can financial security look different from a nine-to-five? Give yourself permission to honor your own truth instead of trying to match someone else's. Break some rules, get creative, and design your own contented life.

DAY 277

Our intuition is connected to our higher Self or the energy of the Universe, so whatever our intuition tells us is always right. We have a tendency to dismiss our intuition because we don't trust it. We have learned to trust the mind but not the body, and our intuition speaks to us through sensation as well as a deep inner knowing. This is not to say I have always been right or always received the outcome I desired. Many times, I thought I was following my intuition when really it was just something I wanted.

How do we strengthen our intuition, our truth, this inner resource? And how do we know the difference between intuition and the mind?

Sometimes, we learn by practice, by screwing up and looking back, realizing where we may not have been honoring our intuition after all. We strengthen our intuition by feeling into sensations in the body, observing the breath, and being present during our practice. Yoga postures heighten intuition because we are in tune with our inner Self. We are less pulled by the mind and all the ways it can mislead us. The more we learn about our mind and what it tells us, the easier it is to discern between mind and inner knowing. Without the distraction of perception, we are able to truly listen and actually hear. Acknowledging inner sensations is integral to your experience and your emotional well-being. When disturbed, you become more skilled at knowing how to realign, how to connect with true Self. Every time you stay with yourself during practice, the subtle differences between mind and intuition become more familiar.

DAY 278

Take a moment to look at yourself in the mirror. Do you see that person? Do you know that person? Do you like that person? Looking at your reflection in the mirror is not an exercise in vanity; it is a beautiful practice in seeing ourselves. Look at yourself in the mirror and acknowledge your goodness. Acknowledge your eyes that have seen and felt so much. Acknowledge your tender parts as well as your wisdom gained. We may never let people see the real us. Can you acknowledge the real you in the mirror?

The part of us people want to see—and the part of us people need—is our truest Self. When we offer our true Self, we offer it all. We don't have to be ashamed of the parts of us that are dark, messy, or full of pain. An accolade we often forget to give ourselves is how much we have been through. We don't recognize the superb accomplishment of pulling ourselves out of a painful experience. We don't recognize the warrior in the mirror. Instead, we often feel slow, behind, or inadequate. Despite all we have carried and all we have overcome, we still feel the need to wish we were different.

Your true Self is more powerful and more beneficial than any fairy-tale story. Your unique path is why people love and adore you. Your gift to the world is who you already are, and it requires no further shaping or fancy bow. Look at that person in the mirror today. That person is deserving, pure of heart, courageous, and wise. That person, in large part because of where you have been, has a lot to share with the world.

DAY 279

Live your truth. How silly to say this because who else's truth would we live? Unfortunately, it's easy to live someone else's truth or behave according to someone else's rules and expectations. Even our expectations of ourselves might not actually be our truth. How do we even access our truth? How do we know what is true for us? According to yoga, the search for our truth is just as meaningful as finding it. On our search for what makes us truly happy and truly ourselves, we probably find out a lot about what we *don't* want. I have little to no interest in gardening, but living in a suburb, gardening is not only a common passion and a pastime but somewhat of an expectation. I used to think something was wrong with me as I watched neighbors spend hours in their gardens, creating colorful beds and pots to catch the eye of those who passed by. I felt obligated to work on my yard—or at least get rid of the unsightly weeds. One day, after several springs of trying to get bulbs to come up and spending money on perennials, I decided to accept that gardening was not for me. I would never have the right system of plants that flowered on schedule and faded just in time for the new blooms to arrive. I had no interest in the effort it took to maintain such a masterpiece. I found plants that required as little attention as possible, and I let go of trying to keep up with the green thumbs of others. Accept your truth. When you don't try to live the truth of someone else, your own truth has space to enter.

DAY 280

"First you do yoga, then yoga does you," my instructor said during a meditation training.

Yoga does you.

When we let go of technique, we open to what wants to happen and what needs to happen instead of manipulating the outcome. Of course there are things we want from our practice, but when we come to our mat with an expectation, we miss the truth of the moment. On our mat, we begin by focusing on technique, the breath, the poses, and the sequence. At some point, technique becomes secondary to what is arriving. The breath may want to expand. A pose may want to take on a different shape. The body may crave rest or faster movement. When we show up to our practice in truth, we are open to what wants to arrive, and we receive everything we need. The gifts of our practice come as a result of our openness and honesty toward the moment, not because we have forced something to occur.

In life, we can show up in truth as well. We show up with equal parts technique and letting go. As we are working toward a dream or accomplishment, we focus on the action of being present rather than what we want the outcome to be. We engage with the practice of showing up so we can recognize the next best action that arrives. Of course we bring our technique, our training, or our expertise to the task at hand, but we also allow for that knowing part of ourselves to step in. We allow for gifts. We allow for letting go. Established in truth, we learn that the moment is more important than the result.

DAY 281

I held on to the fantasy for so long. I longed for the perfect person, family, career, and outside world to make me feel whole, complete, and fulfilled. If I worked hard and got all the pieces right, I wouldn't have to worry about looking within to find happiness or strength. My outer experience would reflect inward, and I would be happy. Outer experience does not necessarily reflect inner contentment. In fact, feeling complete inside and acting from a place of wholeness and authenticity allows everything on the outside to fall into place. And the falling into place for *you* might not look like falling into place for someone else.

Your intention and the foundation you build based on that intention matters. Getting married will not create a loving relationship as much as it will enhance love that is already there. Buying your dream house will bring pride and accomplishment as long as the sole intention is not to fill a void that needs more tending. The path also won't always be easy. It is much harder to do the inner work that brings true, sustainable fulfillment than it is to collect things and people that may bring temporary happiness. Make yourself happy first. Find happiness in the moment, in the circumstance you are in, and from this place of contentment, take actions that support what is already whole, what is already complete. We can expect way too much from the outside image. We expect jobs, people, and possessions to complete us. Nothing will make you complete if you don't first feel complete as you are.

DAY 282

Instead of focusing on society's view, focus on how something makes you feel. We can mistakenly interpret our own feelings according to outside perception. Consider success, for example. Success is often defined according to a monetary amount; when you make a bunch of money, you are a success. But this definition might not be the way *you* feel successful or the qualifier you need in order to be fulfilled. You could spend your entire life chasing someone else's version of success, thinking you need wealth in order to feel successful, instead of determining what success means to you. How do you feel most successful? You may qualify success by lives touched, by projects achieved, or by an event or an adventure. Return to how something makes you feel.

I know I am on the right path when something lights me up. Usually, I feel most alive when I teach someone something. I used to think everyone liked teaching people and everyone got this feeling, but other people may feel most alive when they climb the ladder at a company, when they continue their education, or when they have a family. The thing that makes you feel alive doesn't matter. What matters is that you give yourself permission to define fulfillment according to your own unique definition. When do you feel most like yourself? When does your heart get involved with projects or passions? Who are you with when you feel calm and at ease? We are allowed our own version of success, fulfillment, or any other value. Stay true to yourself by noticing what makes you feel alive.

DAY 283

When I try to force the outer image based on what I think someone wants to see or hear, not only am I being dishonest, but I spend all my energy trying to manage and maintain the appearance. Especially at the beginning of new relationships or friendships, we might be guarded about how much of ourselves we share. We want to put our best foot forward. Eventually though, in order for any meaningful connection to be formed, we must trust that the person we are interacting with can handle the real us. Keeping our guard up will only create turmoil within ourselves and confusion and conflict in the relationship.

When we allow for what is inside us, it won't be for everyone, but it will be perfect for the people who matter—the people who are meant to be in our life and with whom we will form deep bonds. By trying to be the person we think someone wants, we build a rickety, tenuous relationship at best. Likewise, when someone tells you who they are or shares their truth, accept it. Don't think you can change them or dismiss their truth. You will be in more conflict trying to figure each other out than if you had just been honest and accepting from the beginning.

People who are meant to be in your life will be there despite an unattractive past, despite your annoying quirks, and despite the parts you want to hide from. People who love you as you are bring the most fulfilling, meaningful experience. There is no need to waste time and energy trying to be someone else for a relationship that may not even matter.

DAY 284

Truth is so scary. It starts as a whisper, a gentle nudge, and then gets louder, becoming a thought that wakes us up in the middle of the night or a deep knowing that hangs on us throughout our day. *Should we listen?* Often, we hear the truth before we are willing to accept it—and this is okay. Slowly, the truth becomes more apparent until we know we must make a change or do something to honor it. While it's easy to look back and pinpoint the moments we knew, we rarely jump at the truth the second it comes to us. We hear it, and then we push it aside. We do more investigating. We gather more information and run more tests. We want to be sure. Big truths with big consequences are too much to simply turn around on a dime. Of course we are scared when difficult realizations come to light. Even when something is in our best interest long term, it doesn't make it less painful or scary to move forward in the moment. Honoring our truth takes time and trial and error. We probably have to hear the truth many times before we are brave enough to follow through. In the big picture, it doesn't matter how long it takes you to realize the truth. The truth has a way of being very persistent once it has your attention. When the time is right, the truth will be impossible to ignore, and you'll realize you've had enough. You'll move forward with conviction, knowing that the other side must be better than this current place.

DAY 285

"Vulnerability is a strength." Someone said this my first day in rehab, and I wrote it down on a sticky note and taped it to the outside of my binder. I felt like such a failure for needing to go to rehab. I didn't feel sick or mentally ill or vulnerable. I just felt like a jerk and a disappointment. When I got there, the therapists said the bravest thing patients do during their entire treatment is walk through the front door. It's like showing up for the first time, exposed. Vulnerability is a strength. There is no shame in not being perfect. In fact, perfectionism prevents us from being vulnerable. Instead of showing up for ourselves and others as we are, we stay in denial, we lie, we protect, and we cover up. We are too afraid to be the real us, so we exert endless effort in order to not be found out. We try to manage alone and without support. We view our need for support as weakness and our lack of solutions as failure. The times I have been forced to reveal my entire humanness, the imperfect and the messy, are also the times I have learned compassion, forgiveness, and strength. It takes courage to be vulnerable. It takes faith in something bigger to risk one small step into the unknown. As we share pieces of our hidden selves, we are delivered a sense of wholeness and belonging. We are not cast out due to our imperfection but instead rewarded for it. We are fully seen, and this truth heals us like a soft balm. Our vulnerability also heals others, who long to be seen.

DAY 286

We learn early how to gain approval from others, probably parents or caregivers. While there is nothing wrong with wanting to belong or wanting our parents to love us, as we grow up, we can carry the need to be accepted into all our relationships and interactions. We can take on others' emotions when it is not our responsibility. When we constantly seek approval from others, whether parents, partners, or greater society, we are more likely to make decisions that are not in alignment with our core values or our truest Self. Validate yourself: in this moment, place a hand on your heart and a hand on your belly, and say to yourself, "*I see you. I see how hard you are trying. I see all you do.*" Practicing self-validation helps us to unlearn some of the ways we sought approval in the past. It's easy to take on the emotions of others, thinking if we acted differently, spoke differently, or put them ahead of ourselves, we would feel better. Every person has their own responsibility to themselves; it is not our job to carry the emotions of others, even those we love. The behavior of seeking approval does not need to continue into adulthood. As adults, we can begin to recover lost pieces of ourselves that were buried as a result of our need for validation and for love. Today, we can give this love and validation to ourselves. In doing so, we loosen the grip of what someone else wants from us, and we remove the burden of taking on what is not ours to carry. We realize the power of our own validation.

DAY 287

I sat in a recovery circle of fifty people at a weekend retreat. The exercise was to get comfortable accepting compliments. The person next to us had to say something like, "I really loved and appreciated when you _____," filling in the blank, and we had to look the person in the eye and say wholeheartedly, "Thank you. I really like hearing that."

We weren't allowed to shrug our shoulders, roll our eyes, or wave a hand in their direction in order to point out that what we did was no big deal. We couldn't dismiss their compliment; we had to accept it and take it in.

Accepting a compliment is a way of honoring someone else's truth and a way to practice seeing what is true within us. If a compliment makes us uncomfortable, maybe that is our admission. It's vulnerable to receive kind words from others, especially if we weren't trying to do anything in the first place. For me, some of the most difficult compliments to accept are the ones that come as a result of me just being myself. Without effort, my natural way had an effect. It's a bit ironic when we spend so much energy trying to get people to like us, and yet when we hear a compliment, we push it away. We want to honor everyone's truth, and that includes words that are spoken to us. We can practice receiving compliments gracefully, without detracting from them. Hold compliments like a soft embrace. Let them settle in and be acknowledged. The person took the time to say it to you because you had an impact. We really do affect others by being our most authentic Self.

DAY 288

The Gospel of Thomas offers a bold statement about honoring our truth. It says, "If you bring forth what is within you, what you bring forth will save you. If you do not bring forth what is within you, what you do not bring forth will destroy you."[58] This quote always makes me slightly unsettled. *Really?* Not bringing forth my truth will destroy me? Connecting this quote to the practice of satya, I interpret it as having two points. First, there is a unique gift that resides within each of us. Second, we should not be afraid of or doubt this unique gift. In fact, we should lean into our gifts and do whatever it takes to bring them forth. This quote tells me that not only should I honor my truth, but I am responsible for bringing it out—my fulfillment and my purpose to the world seem to depend on this.

You *can* allow what is within you to come to the surface. You *can* honor that hobby, passion, career choice, or pastime. We don't have to feel irresponsible or indulgent for living our truth. Actually, it is the way we serve. Take a moment to notice how much time you spend each day honoring an activity that you know is your gift. If you feel you have no gifts, consider what you enjoy doing. Doing activities simply because they make us happy is a perfectly acceptable and essential practice. Your gift does not have to change the world. But somehow, by making yourself happy, by doing things that honor who you are, others benefit. It's a win-win.

....
58. Pagels, "The Gospel of Thomas."

DAY 289

To be grounded in your truth also means to take responsibility. This might seem scary at first, but once you take responsibility for all the parts of your life, even the mistakes, you also get to take pride in all the successes. We live in a society that emphasizes perfect paths and misses out on the blessings that are in the supposed setbacks. How do you change the story of your past? By accepting it, by letting go of shame, and by knowing it was needed in order to get you here.

Every experience holds a lesson along your path. The path to knowing the true Self takes some pain and some regret. It is possible to acknowledge the truth of your past, even unpleasant situations, as part of what grew you into something new. Taking responsibility for our past doesn't always feel good. I do not like to look back on moments in my life when I was unhealthy, disturbed, or unaware. But disowning my truth, burying unsightly parts of my experience, keeps me in regret and shame. It also keeps me in denial about how these parts of myself brought me where I am today—more aware, more conscious, and more capable. Our truth does not need to be perfect. We can accept our whole Self as a work in progress and as a teacher along the way. Look to the truth of today. *Are you taking responsibility? Are you honoring your accomplishments?*

Through a series of errors, we finally might be able to look back and see that all those wrong turns were actually blessings. Then we may justifiably wonder, *"What blessings are happening today that I am mistaking for flaws?"*

DAY 290

The only way to not be in a constant battle with the Self is to allow who you really are to emerge—regardless of contradictions or even offensiveness. I believe the best parts about humanity are the experiences we share in order to connect and the individual differences that bring new viewpoints to the same experience. Everyone's individual truth brings more richness and depth to the collective experience. We all get to own our experience, and everyone's perspective can be true. We are taught in terms of A/B, either/or, and right/wrong. Really, there are infinite answers, and they all depend on who you are and where you came from. It's impossible to determine one person's truth from someone else's reality. If we had their experience and their life, we'd believe and act the same way they do. Understanding that beneath our individual experiences we are all the same allows us to have more compassion and understanding, even for those we dislike.

We get intimidated by differences; we may judge or feel inadequate. We wonder how to relate to people who are not like us. We may try to mold or change in order to appear more like them. The most impressive act is to be authentic. The parts of a person that are the most interesting and bring the most gifts are those that are a result of their unique experience. Having compassion for your own experience—and everyone else's—helps you to show up more fully and confidently as you are. You are individually, extraordinarily, and perfectly you.

DAY 291

What is true? What is real? We always bring our practice back to these questions. Asking what is true is to dive deep into the inquiry of rediscovering ourselves and asking who we really are, not from yesterday or even ten minutes ago but right now—in this moment.

The Sutras say when we practice truth, honesty follows us and becomes our true nature.[59] When the mind is clear, not affected by false narrative, we arrive at a place of truth. It's easy to drag false narrative into present experience. I can be at a social event and be completely unpresent. Worried about something in my mind, I can't enjoy myself. If truth is our true nature, then we are most content when living in our authentic experience. As soon as I notice I am lost in story, it's helpful for me to focus on something happening right in front of me—a conversation, a sight, sound, or smell. I can acknowledge the worry without letting it overtake my experience, especially if there is nothing I can do about it. Once I realize I am in my mind, I can bring myself back to the situation at hand and my anxiety lessens.

We stray from our truth on a regular basis. As the mind runs, we get pulled into old story or false belief. We must constantly adjust and come back to ourselves. This is the importance of our practice, to tune in to what is real in the moment. Just like we can notice the mind wander in our practice, we can observe it wandering in other experiences as well. There is always the opportunity and choice to take a breath and bring yourself back to right here.

....
59. Satchidananda, *The Yoga Sutras of Patanjali*, 124.

DAY 292

Saying our truth out loud is scary and takes guts. In relationships, an ideal situation is when we voice our needs or feelings and our partner responds with compassion and understanding. But sometimes, when we admit our truth, we are met with challenge, criticism, or blame. If the other person constantly questions or twists your truth, you may have learned to stay quiet in order to avoid conflict. Believing our truth regardless of what others think, especially those we love, takes deep awareness and trust in ourselves. We may not even need the other person to do anything; just hearing our truth can be enough.

If a partner or loved one responds to your feelings with invalidation, you might try to manipulate your truth by telling yourself you don't really feel that way. You may minimize your feelings in order to avoid further hurt. This invalidation, by ourselves and our partner, only covers the problem and leads to no growth or resolution. Even if the issue is brushed over in the moment, it will probably show up again in a different scenario. Your needs are valid, and they can be expressed without attacking or blaming the other person. Stating our truth doesn't always bring the results or the reaction we want, but it does lead to more truth about the relationship. If the other person isn't willing to meet us halfway, we may need to make another choice. Honesty in any relationship has the capacity to deepen the connection through understanding and compassion. State your truth lovingly and assertively. When we share our truth without attack and with the intention to heal and grow, we honor ourselves as well as the relationship.

DAY 293

Comparison is a clever way to avoid our own truth or not discover it at all. Comparing to others also leads to poor choices, choices that are not necessarily in our best interest. In yoga, we might risk injury by doing a pose that is too challenging for our ability. In life, we might try to attain an image or an outer appearance while sacrificing what we really want. Constantly, for the sake of comparing, we overdo, overwork, and overextend. We risk our own values and our own safety in order to fill the void of feeling less than. Feeling inadequate makes us act on fear: fear of being different, fear of not getting something, or fear of doing something the wrong way. Comparing makes us competitive when there is plenty of room for all versions of beauty, success, and happiness.

I easily know when I am in comparing-mode. My brain is racing, unable to focus, and I can't stop feeding the stories I am telling myself. We are so conditioned to fall for the lie that we are not good enough or that someone else knows something we don't. I might see someone who has a life or career I want, but that doesn't mean I have to be exactly like them. That doesn't mean there is anything wrong with my way.

Honoring your own truth is more important than trying to match your life or your choices to someone else's. Let go of what someone else's relationship, career, or outer image looks like. Ask what will work for you and your own contentment today. No one is watching you except you.

DAY 294
Third Eye Practice

Ajna is the sixth chakra, also called the third eye, which is located at the forehead's center, and represents our inner guru. This chakra connects us to our wisdom center and truth. Activating the third eye stimulates the pituitary gland, which controls hormones and regulates body functions. The third eye controls our perception. According to *The Language of Yin*, with it, "we get clarity, wisdom, and intuition, and we can view life through the eyes of the soul."[60] When this chakra is blocked, we may have trouble making decisions. We overanalyze. We're closed in our thinking and way of seeing situations. Practices that open the third eye bring more clarity to our experience. We are open to new perspectives and ideas. We learn to connect with our inner guru to make choices that reflect our core values and honor our truth. We learn to trust ourselves.

Lie on your belly with elbows bent and hands stacked on top of one another. Rest your forehead on your hands and close your eyes. Wiggle your hips. Relax your legs. Notice the sensation of pressure on the center of your forehead. Gently rock your head from side to side, massaging this area. Allow your jaw and facial muscles to soften. Observe the skin and the lips; let everything in the face be heavy. With eyes closed, draw your attention to the spot above and between your eyes. Gaze here. Notice any shapes, colors, or messages. Trust that this practice is working and your intuition is strengthening.

....
60. Harris, *The Language of Yin*, 162–63.

DAY 295

We are the only ones who know ourselves so wholly and completely that when we abandon ourselves, it hurts. Something deep inside begs us to change course. The anxiety of forgetting who we are fills our stomach and our heart. A heaviness sits inside our chest, and we have to gently ask what it means. If you've ever felt unsettled, uneasy, or a bit anxious in general, it may be because you have stepped away from your truth.

Often, we mistake the uneasy feeling as someone else's fault or related to an outside circumstance. We may look around and start to analyze how others could change or what we could shift on the outside in order to make ourselves feel better. However, that nagging sensation of unease is completely within us to resolve. What have we done to step away from our truth? Are we living someone else's life or someone else's view of who we should be? Are we relying on other people for validation and therefore acting in a way that goes against what we really want?

Instead of trying to master people or circumstance, strive to live in a way that honors you at your center. Get used to listening to your body and not accepting the inner voice as crazy or unwise. As a result, watch everything else around you fall into place—your relationships, your career, your day-to-day life. The Universe will conspire in your favor as long as you are on your path, and when you're not, your body tells you pretty quickly. You get sick, tired, or frustrated. Listen. Pay attention. You know yourself better than anyone, and your body usually knows before you do.

DAY 296

Move from your center—in yoga and in life. On our mat, we focus a lot on our core. A strong core helps our body move with integrity. We are better able to balance, to transition, and to avoid injury. Moving from a strong center and an integrated core gives us options and possibilities. Poses become accessible. Balance becomes more easeful. Sitting can be done for longer periods of time without discomfort. Our center helps us physically but also emotionally. The stillness and introspection quiets outside noise and brings us back to our truth. Time on the mat is time to reflect without others' input or opinions. We practice moving from our center in a pose so we can act with the same level of integrity in life. Telling lies no longer feels good, so it becomes less of an option or a default. Treating the body unkindly starts to feel violent or pushy, so we are more likely to practice self-love off the mat as well. Strengthening and toning muscles in our core gives us a defined, powerful center—one we can feel. We stand taller, physically and mentally. We make better decisions. We trust ourselves. Above all, we are honest, and we take responsibility. We can sleep at night, no longer disrupted by living a life that is not true to who we are. When someone comes to me with doubt, shame, or low self-esteem, we always start by building core strength. We find balance and engage muscles in mountain pose. Feel your strength on the mat so you can step into your power in life. Today, move from your center. Stand strong in your truth.

DAY 297

Satya continually asks us to seek answers from within. From our own place of truth, we become masters of our experience, whether that involves another person or situation or an issue within ourselves. So easily we get caught up in the material world, both out of fear and a need to feel fulfilled. We expect people to behave a certain way, and we become very flustered when they don't. Our culture is based on systems of reciprocity. We get paid in exchange for labor, we trade money for goods and services, and we give birthday gifts, expecting that the recipients will reciprocate. I'm not saying we should do away with these exchanges or expectations, but we can return to the practice of being fulfilled from within in order to place less pressure on the outside world and more ownership on ourselves. Everything you seek is already within you. The truth of who you are is rooted in a power that comes from within. By cultivating this resource, we learn that we are loved despite someone's actions, and we are whole despite our circumstance. Our motivation to engage in our spiritual practice is selfless; we have no expectation of gain but are open to receive the gifts that are meant for us—gifts such as inner peace, calmness, patience, and abiding faithfulness. When we are disturbed, we know we can ask for solutions within our own heart instead of relying on someone else. Over time, our practice chips away at fear and ego, and we become less selfish. This small shift in our being ripples out to everyone we touch and everything we do.

DAY 298

I want to believe that I can let go the ugly, self-absorbed, unbecoming parts of me, never to let them surface again. But without our shadow, there is no light. Without our unbecoming qualities, we would not have the opposite. I admire patience. I try to emulate this quality as a parent, a daughter, and a partner. I can practice patience successfully, but I can also be very impatient, not understanding, and frantic. We are all both—the shadow and the light. Our greatest assets can also be our worst liabilities. Qualities we admire might also be aspects of ourselves we want to make progress on. Rather than pretend we are beyond our flaws and triggers, we can see them, acknowledge them, accept them, and shift our perspective.

As parents, lovers, children, and friends, we are never perfect. Those closest to us often experience our unruly Self because we allow them to see the real us. In his book *Owning Your Own Shadow*, Robert Johnson writes, "To own one's shadow is to reach a holy place—an inner center—not attainable in any other way."[61] In your center is a beautiful, tender place, a place that longs to be acknowledged and not hidden or denied. In your center lies truth, not the front you put on for the rest of the world. When your shadow side emerges, when something you have been working on comes out anyway, own it. Owning your shadow lights up some of the darkness. By accepting every part of ourselves, we give the dark and scary parts a little less power.

....
61. Johnson, *Owning Your Own Shadow*, 17.

DAY 299

I thought not breaking in the first place would be easier than trying to put all the pieces back together, or at least I could hide the filled-in cracks and glued-together shards. Letting it all show would be disastrous. Because of that belief, I had two rules in life:

1. Don't break; you'll never be the same.
2. Collect things and people that will complete you.

Looking at these rules today, I think I really underestimated myself. If we don't break, we never realize our own strength, and we never grow. If we rely on others to complete us, we give all our power away, and we never get to discover who we are. There's an idea I love about gathering our scattered pieces that relates so well to truth. When we start to get curious about who we are, when we start to follow own our path and take responsibility for our experience, we collect all the parts of ourselves that we've lost and tried so desperately to keep hidden. We take back our power. Instead of relying on someone else to fix us, we own ourselves fully. Instead of hiding, we arrive. We learn to accept ourselves, forgive ourselves, and take care of ourselves—maybe for the first time. Not only does breaking open add more beauty to our journey, but breaking open makes us whole. The things I was most afraid to face and reveal are the exact things that would complete me. Breaking makes you whole by bringing you the gifts of your own path, by allowing you to realize your own strength, and by showing you all the ways you underestimate yourself.

DAY 300

Emotions are not always true. Children react to their emotions as truth by screaming, throwing something, or acting based on any feeling that arrives. As we grow into adults and develop the ability to interpret our emotions, we learn self-control and self-regulation. We are able to watch an emotion arrive and determine its relevance. Neuroscience says the brain has both a "top-down" and "bottom-up" effect. Top-down happens when we bring a topic or situation to mind and it elicits an emotion. Likewise, we can have an emotion and the sensation creates thoughts about a person or situation; this is bottom-up.[62] While we often can't control emotions that arrive, we have a choice in how we see things. If our intention is anger, that emotion will be manifested in our experience, like a bad mood sabotaging out day. Choosing a positive emotion helps to produce more positive interactions.

While we want to acknowledge our emotions, we have a choice to reflect on our sensations and decide how to respond. Expectations of how our day will unfold or how a scenario will play out are powerful. We have power over our experience by the emotions we bring into it. If there is a situation that truly makes you anxious, avoid it. When discomfort arrives in a somewhat neutral experience, notice and see if you can adjust your mindset and therefore your emotional response.

....
62. Tomaino, *Awakening the Brain*, 124.

DAY 301

I wore pretty dresses to church and on holidays because my parents wanted me to, and it was what all the other little girls did. Seeing the approval on my parents' faces meant the world to me. My sister complained and rallied against the dresses, like most things my parents asked her to do. I wondered why she made such a big deal; let's just smile and do what's expected, and no one will bother us.

Into adulthood, I continued playing the part instead of developing my own sense of what made me happy. My truth got very blurry. Who was I? When we get out of alignment with our true Self, when we have forgotten to acknowledge our own wants and needs, there is an overwhelming sense that we don't belong. We have no feeling of "home" in our soul because we are always playing a part. I knew I was addicted long before I decided to quit. I knew I had an eating disorder, but I would never admit it. I feared if anyone found out the real me, they wouldn't like me anymore.

If you look at the person in the mirror and they are not who you intended, maybe it's time for a realignment. Maybe there is a need or a desire you can answer. Maybe you are acting one way despite it feeling untrue for you. We feel a sense of home and belonging when we behave in a way that honors our soul. Find the truth inside yourself and enact relentless, compassionate, all-encompassing love for that person. Everyone who loves you will love you even more, and they'd love to see you return home.

DAY 302

Uncovering the big truths about who we are and how we operate takes some intense effort at first. In the beginning, it may seem like the changes are impossible and time consuming. Like any practice, the initial effort feels clunky and maybe daunting, but as we get accustomed to the new routine, we find that the process doesn't require as much thought or intense focus. We naturally treat the body with more kindness, craving healthy foods and practicing compassionate self-care. We more easily say "no" when needed and don't let emotions build up and fester. Our new way of life becomes just that—a way of life. That doesn't mean we don't slip back to old, comfortable ways. Practicing satya does not mean we are perfect from here on out. Practicing satya means we get more accustomed to self-awareness. We know when we are dishonoring ourselves or our emotions. We know when we are acting out untruths, and it doesn't feel so good. We adjust as needed; we take care of life and relationships as we go, and we don't create such an overwhelming mess or crisis. Once we shift a belief and embark on a new behavior, we remain faithful and committed to our practice. The goal is not to be perfect but to recognize old patterns as they arrive. Once we start practicing truthfulness and see all the ways we were hiding, manipulating, or denying ourselves, we seek our authentic Self above all else. We love who we are, and we're proud of where we've been. We are not afraid of the truth because we see the benefits of living an honest life, a life that reflects our gifts, our progress, and our whole Self.

PRACTICE 11
Unconditional Love

Once we understand our oneness, our connection to all beings, the world becomes softer, more beautiful, and more
heartbreaking. Unconditional love means we have complete acceptance of Self and everyone else. We practice nonviolence, or ahimsa,
the first of the five yamas. Practicing unconditional love doesn't
mean we don't stand up for our beliefs or our convictions or don't
want change, but we do let go of judgment in order to see truth. We
know that we all are shaped by experience, so everyone is behaving
as best they know how. If we had their experiences, we may act and
think the same as them. We shift our gaze from critique and self-
righteousness to one of understanding. We let go of self-serving
ways and focus on how we can benefit others. We stay open despite
pain, and we always strive to lead from the heart.

DAY 303

Love drives out fear. Fear arrives as thoughts and stories in the mind, and the solution is not to dismiss the fear or fight with it but to add more love. Consider times you have felt judgmental, frustrated, impatient, confused, or agitated. When we shut out love and understanding, when we close our hearts, fear has an easy way in. Fear tells us we are right, justified, and superior or that we are unworthy, incapable, and dumb. Fear takes hold of our mind and our thoughts. We ruminate about our circumstance or whatever is bothering us. It is impossible to let go because we are high on the self-righteousness or the self-wallowing. Let love step in.

Recognize that you are behaving out of fear and that the mind has you caught in an illusion. You don't need to push out the fear. Instead, love that part of yourself that is fearful. Acknowledge the hurt, and acknowledge your desire to figure this all out with your mind. Then, step back and add more love. Ways to add love can be to meditate, do yoga, or go for a walk. Take a bath or make yourself a healthy meal. Call a friend and offer to help. Try to stay out of the mind's desire to keep you in fear. Place a hand on your heart and remember who you are. See if something inside you shifts. See if you move a little closer to love. When we do yoga or meditate, when we return to the breath, we remember that we are more than our mind. We return to the divine, loving part of ourselves, and as our awareness shifts, so does our heart.

DAY 304

Ahimsa means "nonviolence," and it is the first of the five yamas in the Eight Limbs of Yoga. Of all the limbs, nonviolence starts everything off. Many yoga philosophers and practicing yogis believe that nonviolence is the foundation and the core of the entire practice of yoga. I've even heard that if you truly practiced this one principle, there would be no need for the rest. Imagine a world where everyone practiced nonviolence all the time. Our experience would be very different.

Ahimsa refers to how we treat others, the earth, and ourselves. Without this practice, it is difficult to achieve anything else. What does practicing nonviolence look like? We tend to think of violence as physical, such as war, fighting, and abuse. Yes, these are all acts of violence. However, most of us do not engage in this type of physical violence. Violence, according to yoga, goes way beyond physical. Violence includes how we treat ourselves and talk to ourselves, as well as what we expect from others. Once we start exploring nonviolence beyond the physical, we see how acting violently plays a large role in our life.

Often, the most violent acts we commit are against ourselves. We have an ugly, nasty critical voice that emerges, even when something good is happening. We operate from this critical voice instead of our hearts. We allow fear, doubt, and low self-confidence to rule. We compare ourselves to others, we feel like we are not enough, and we refuse to forgive ourselves for mistakes in our past. All of this is violence. Let's begin the undoing and a new way of treating ourselves with more kindness.

DAY 305

The practice of nonviolence is so big and complex, it affects almost every part of our life. To practice nonviolence 100 percent of the time would be impossible—never being critical, never harming, never polluting. So, what do we do with this practice of ahimsa? Do we give up? Do we stop trying? Of course not. Practicing nonviolence teaches us so much about ourselves and how we operate. Practicing nonviolence teaches us about humanity and our purpose. Practicing nonviolence teaches us how to *love*.

In the spirit of nonviolence, remember that cultivating awareness of how we think, feel, or behave is never meant to bring about guilt, shame, or bad feelings about ourselves. Awareness is the first step to helping us adopt a healthier way of being. So, if you have noticed a few ways you might have been unloving toward yourself, all of it is an opportunity to treat yourself more kindly.

Here are some journal prompts to explore nonviolence:

+ How has your definition of nonviolence expanded? What does it now include?
+ What are some ways you have noticed you harm yourself? What would acting with more kindness look like?
+ What are some ways you notice you are harmful toward others? Do you harm others by judging, criticizing, or thinking you know what's best for them?
+ Finally, acknowledge all the ways you practice loving-kindness to yourself and others. Be proud of the ways you already and naturally demonstrate love.

DAY 306

Fear sneaks up on us. We might think we are honoring our heart when we are actually running the other direction. Fear wants immediate results, while intuition is trusting and patient. Fear does not want you to take a big inhale, pause, and relax. Fear wants you to cling, grasp, and panic.

Fear can drown not only romantic relationships but also friendships, business ventures, creative pursuits, exercise goals, and money matters. Fear holds you hostage inside a constant cycle of nothing feeling good enough so you will always be chasing. Moving toward love does not feel like a fight or a conquest. When you move toward love, you feel centered without the anxiety of lack or loss. There is no hurry, no fear of missing out or being late. When you lean into love, more love is sent back to you, maybe in the form of helpers or opportunities. Love manifests more love. We're so used to acting out of fear, we might reach for instant gratification instead of abiding trust, but that reward is fleeting, and it will not produce long-term results. Leaning into love presents ideas, paths, and people that once seemed out of reach. Leaning into love makes the best relationships and partnerships even better. Set your intention and your compass toward love. Sit down to breathe instead of reacting. Give yourself some space and some time so you don't feed the fear and so you can make the next right choice. Check in because fear tries to derail us. After enough practice, choosing love will come more naturally, and you'll notice a shift in your demeanor. You'll realize that honoring yourself in love will actually bring the best outcome.

DAY 307
Loving-Kindness Meditation

Begin seated. Close your eyes. Observe your breath. After a moment, bring to mind someone you love dearly. This person can be alive or no longer with you. Hold their image in your mind's eye, and let their presence fill you with love. Say these words out loud or in your head, "I wish you peace. I wish you health. I wish you a life of ease." Send them love.

Next, bring to mind an acquaintance. Maybe a neighbor you don't really talk to. Maybe the person you see at the coffee shop or the store. Hold the image of this person in your mind and in your heart. Repeat the phrases, "I wish you peace. I wish you health. I wish you a life of ease." Send them love.

Bring to mind someone you have a challenging relationship with. Keep the challenge small but not insignificant. Maybe someone at work or someone with whom you just don't see eye to eye. Notice sensations that arise when you think of this challenging person. Repeat the same phrases to them, "I wish you peace. I wish you health. I wish you a life of ease." Send them love.

Now place your hand on your own heart, and say to yourself, "I wish you peace. I wish you health. I wish you a life of ease. I wish you peace. I wish you health. I wish you a life of ease. I wish you peace. I wish you health. I wish you a life of ease." Send yourself love. When ready, come back to your body and feel any shifts in sensation or perception. When you feel like the meditation is complete, open your eyes.

DAY 308

When we get hurt, we jump to our own defense, and judgment, anger, and fear arrive. It's hard to seek awareness and understanding of the other person, but this is precisely what love asks us to do. Feeling hurt is a sensation, a gripping tightness in the chest or a punch in our gut. It's helpful to feel and observe the physical sensations of any hurt because sensations are real and keep us present. Once the mind is involved, ego and fear quickly take over; we are no longer focused on the current hurt and are instead reliving everything from the past. Old wounds and ideas are navigating the experience, and we have lost focus on the current sensation of pain.

We can heal a hurt without involving the person who caused us pain. We can observe the sensation and look toward our own heart to uncover what this pain is here to teach us. Don't jump to conclusions right away; feel your pain, allow it to move, and then decide on the next best action.

When communication in a relationship is necessary, we want to express ourselves clearly and without attack. Focus on your feelings but don't assume the motives of the other person. Any meaningful relationship requires communication in order to be understood and to understand. Misunderstanding is an opportunity to learn more about ourselves and those we care about. It might not look like much, but those who observe their pain in order to gain the highest understanding are abiding warriors. With greater awareness of our emotions, communication becomes a moment in truly hearing one another.

DAY 309

In Sanskrit, the word *karuna* translates to "compassion" and "self-compassion." When we practice love, let's include ourselves. Compassion also relates to our practice of ahimsa (nonviolence). Ahimsa asks us to practice nonviolence to ourselves as well as others. There are many ways we harm ourselves unintentionally or treat ourselves with little compassion. When it comes to love and nonviolence, in addition to how we view and treat others, we also want to explore ways we are violent or uncompassionate with ourselves through critical self-talk, unreasonable expectations, unforgiveness, and a lack of self-acceptance. Accepting yourself exactly as you are is a huge demonstration of love. Accepting yourself instead of blaming yourself, berating yourself, or hating yourself is the opposite of violence and the definition of self-compassion. Where are we critical? How can we be more understanding? Are we hard on ourselves? Can we practice forgiveness and grace?

When I decided to forgive myself for my past, my regrets, and, most importantly, the harmful ways I treated my body, I wept. I cried for that unloved girl and unaccepted woman. She deserved so much more.

You deserve so much love, and you can start right now.

DAY 310

I love without fear. I love without bounds. I love even though I have been hurt. I love and know I am always loved.

Our hearts close. For various reasons and circumstances—and because it is a natural response to threat—our hearts close. We forget the joy and fulfillment that come from walking this Earth with an open heart. We are more comfortable in the longing, unwilling to risk any pain or discomfort. Here is a secret about love. We do not need any person, circumstance, or outcome in order to experience love. To experience love, we only need an open heart. We do not need a perfect relationship or a soulmate. We do not need our dream career. What does an open heart look like, feel like, and act like? An open heart leaps to help a stranger. An open heart stands in awe of the moving clouds and a painted sunset. An open heart asks, *"What can I offer?"* instead of *"What can I gain?"*

There are small ways to wiggle a heart open. Little by little, we may experience the wonder of our existence. Something makes you smile or laugh. You have a moment of feeling like everything is going to be all right. Often after yoga or meditation, I feel a complete shift in my nature because my heart has just opened as a result of the poses and attention on my breath. We step away lighter, and our problems seem less acute. An open heart behaves with no conditions, no resentments, no grudges, and no payback. An open heart swells at the idea of giving love and does not seek anything in return.

DAY 311
Heart Openers

Consider your heart in yoga postures that ask you to open. On an inhale, lift your heart space and notice your chest expand. While in triangle pose, keep your chest turned sideways, rather than letting it drop towards the ground. In a twist, broaden your shoulders and expand with the breath.

Poses that let us reach our sternum forward, tilt our heart open, or breathe into the space behind the ribs are not only excellent for posture, but they also help us behave from a place of love and understanding in life. As your heart space lifts, your shoulders drop into alignment. As you follow your heart, life brings you what you need. There is much more to following our heart than adopting a fantastical, optimistic outlook. Following our heart doesn't mean everything looks pretty. Following our heart means making difficult, often painful choices. Following our heart looks like ending a relationship, setting a firm boundary, telling someone how we feel, telling someone goodbye, or moving forward through fear and self-doubt.

Following our heart can mean loss, heartache, vulnerability, courage, and risk. But following our heart will always lead us down the path to our own peace and contentment. Following our heart will lead us to love—love for ourselves or for someone else. Following our heart will lead us to our true purpose, whether it's a career, passion, or deep healing. Following our heart is different from reacting to every emotional whim. When we follow our heart, we acknowledge a place from deep within. It is a pure, loving place that always has our best interests.

DAY 312

To feel love, we need to give it. To be understood, we need to understand. These suggestions are repeated in ancient yogic texts, many religions, and all twelve-step recovery programs. The Prayer of Saint Francis echoes the intention with "Grant that I may not so much seek to be consoled as to console, to be understood as to understand, to be loved as to love."[63]

Regardless of practices or beliefs, the common thread is love. Love for all beings. Love for ourselves. Love for the agony and the awakening. The answer to every problem and every pain point is love. So, what's so hard about it? Why do we so often rail against love?

We mistake love as something that keeps score. We label people, including ourselves, as deserving or undeserving. We feel love is earned, so we try desperately to behave in ways that will make people love us. We feel unworthy, and we push love away. We hold back our own love, and we use it against people. We try to control it. Love does not have to be so complicated or scary. With practice, as we put ourselves out there, we notice people who will catch us. We see who shows up. We show up for ourselves. The excitement of an open heart starts to feel like a strength rather than a weakness. Giving love—acting in love—brings us a spiritual experience right here on Earth. Being closed off and keeping score no longer feels comfortable. Just go for it. Wherever you have been holding back, let your heart open, and trust that the people, gifts, and lessons you will receive are worth it.

....
63. "Peace Prayer of Saint Francis."

DAY 313

I used to think I was just independent and strong-willed, but I've learned that a guarded heart, masked as independence, might be what kept me feeling alone in the world. We need people. Humans require connection, someone to listen and to sit by our side. To feel connection, we must share something vulnerable and real. The more façades we put up, the less others are able to see us, which is exactly what we so desperately need; we need to be seen, to be heard.

Protecting myself from pain became more important than putting my true Self out there. I gave people the version they wanted and basically stayed guarded from any real emotion, any connection, and any risk of disappointment. I never asked for help—not with the kids or with juggling life. The first time I felt desperate enough to admit I couldn't do something on my own was with my addiction. Recovery meetings became so much more than a tool to stop drinking. Somehow, by listening to others share their stories, stories that were just like mine, I felt seen. I felt heard. I also felt safe, like I could actually be myself, even though the parts of myself I was sharing were so dark and imperfect.

Revealing our imperfections, in any relationship or community, is how we let others in. The protection I had been wearing may have been padding me from pain, but it was also keeping me isolated and alone. Trying to do everything on my own kept everyone at an arm's length. I learned that by showing up as my imperfect Self, I received the love and connection I had always desired.

DAY 314

I always thought praying or asking for divine support had to happen with something or someone outside myself, like a person in the sky with a robe and a gavel. I've learned that my own heart is my lifeline and connection to the Divine. My heart somehow knows exactly what I need, even when I don't want to hear it. My heart yearns to be acknowledged. My own self-abandonment has caused much more heartbreak than what anyone else has ever done to me. When I haven't followed my intuition, when I've ignored my heart despite its pleas, I've felt more of a loss than the outside event. When I realize I have gone against my own heart, it hurts.

So, what does it look like to lead with your heart?

Place a hand there—right over your heart. Feeling your own heart is like acknowledging yourself for the first time. We are conditioned to think we do not matter. We are conditioned to suck it up, ignore ourselves, and wear a smile. If your heart is broken, admit it. If your heart is overjoyed, celebrate. If your heart is longing, ask what it needs. Asking your own heart is like asking the Divine for help; our heart has been our own personal genie beating inside our chest this entire time, not just to keep us alive but to help us thrive. After a lifetime relying on practicality and approval, it's difficult to trust our own intuition and feelings. With practice, you get better at it. With practice, you learn that everything you need has been right there inside you. Everything you need is there—under your hand and inside your own heart.

DAY 315
Sphinx Pose

Lie on your belly with legs extended behind you and rest on your elbows, like a child watches TV. Press your palms and forearms into the mat, keeping your arms parallel. Lower your shoulders away from your ears and let your lower jaw instinctively drop. Breathe. Observe your ribs expand as you inhale. Watch your collarbones lift. Now pull back on your elbows and forearms as if trying to move the mat. Reach your sternum forward. Visualize your heart space shining ahead. Keep your chin parallel to the earth or your gaze looking down at your mat.

Sphinx pose is a heart opener. It also lengthens the spine and tones the low back. To protect the low back, keep focusing on the heart reaching forward and engaging the muscles in the low back rather than coming up too high by pressing into the arms and elbows. To direct your heart outward, utilize the muscles in your core and low back. Find the balance between the heart reaching and the low back toning. Observe any tightening of unnecessary muscles or resistance to the pose. Often, I feel most comfortable with my heart in a closed position, like forward fold, where I can relax and curve the spine. I feel the weight of gravity like a warm blanket, reminding me I can simply let go, simply be. Remaining with my heart open takes effort; muscles spring into action and engage. In order to keep my heart reaching forward in sphinx, my core and my back need to be strong. Little by little, the more you practice sphinx, muscles in your low back will tone in order to better support your heart shining ahead.

DAY 316

Regardless of outside circumstance, other people's behaviors, or any exterior view, you are—at your core—still you. There is a light that forever exists inside you, even when you don't feel like shining, even when you don't feel like you have anything else to give, and even when you don't feel so bright. This is the part of you that remains abiding in love, believing with your whole heart that good exists and joy is accessible, even when the world crashes and roils all around you. In everyday moments, in breaths, in mealtimes and bedtimes, in hugs and in handshakes, light exists. The love at the center of the Universe is the same love that beats inside your heart.

Stephen Cope describes beings who embody this calm center as a "home base" for those who are suffering.[64] Everyday people, who have no training and no technique, simply beat with the heart of all beings to hold us up and to keep us safe when we need to remember. An outside event can shake us into unknowing and despair, but the kindness and generosity of others carry us through, like a boat that keeps frothing waters at bay, and deliver us to shore. Even in difficult times, remember that the person you have always been exists inside of you. Moments that deliver us to presence, moments that are so rich with pain we are forced to take stock in what is good, allow us to stop our rushing ahead and focus instead on the small gifts of right now. You are always loved, no matter who hurts you. You are always supported, no matter how alone you feel. Look for your home base.

....
64. Cope, *Yoga and the Quest for the True Self*, 152.

DAY 317

"When you meet anyone, remember it is a holy encounter."[65] This quote from A Course in Miracles means every interaction and every relationship, however fleeting or seemingly pointless, has great purpose. The holy encounter is the idea that every person has a predestined reason for existing. Every person you meet and each lifelong relationship are all fate, and they exist to teach you something along your spiritual journey. The person at the gas station and your spouse both qualify as holy encounters. We don't always know who has a lasting effect on us, and we also may not know or fully understand the effect we have on others.

For many relationships, we know who our people are. You know the people who have come into your life for a period of time and affected you to your core. They changed you. Maybe they hurt you. Maybe they loved you. But after the encounter, you emerged a different version of yourself.

The best shift in perspective that comes from believing in the concept of the holy encounter is that we are suddenly free. Relationships are no longer tied to an image or outcome; there is no such thing as a failed relationship. Holy encounters don't need vows or ceremonies. Holy encounters can happen in an instant. We exist to help every person, and every person exists to help us. Every relationship is a holy encounter. Every human being is your fate and here to teach you something.

....
65. Schucman and Thetford, A Course in Miracles, 150.

DAY 318

There is a physics to the Universe, a vibration to every cell and every object. Trees, humans, other animals, and music all vibrate differently to create their form. Love is said to be the highest vibration of all, and I believe this because when I have felt pure love, everything around me seems more vibrant, noticeable, and real. The vibration of love is so high, it nearly drops me to my knees. Sometimes, love is a sensation when we are in child's pose or a knowing as we stare behind closed eyes. Love is beyond rational thought, and we can access it through the body—through keen observation. When I truly allow myself to accept the vibration of love, it's hard to take a full breath in. I wriggle beneath the weight of love's fullness.

To connect with the vibration of love, think of a person you adore—a grandmother, a caregiver, a teacher—someone who emanates love regardless of the pain and suffering of life. Let that feeling wash over you. Even though you are not physically with that person, you are creating the same experience in energy.

Feel this energy. Let the love consume you until you beat with the same vibration as the trees, the clouds, and the ocean. I believe that anything is possible here because your body is singing with the truth of who you are. Love exists whether we touch it or not. Whenever I have these experiences, they are fleeting. We glimpse love, and then we quickly forget. We come back to our work, our life, and our problems, but for those moments, when we vibrate with love and remember we are divine, we have hope.

DAY 319

Our version of what we deserve and what is possible is so limiting. The love of the Universe wants us to remember our greatness so we don't block all that is in store for us. Maybe it feels corny or selfish to love yourself, but when we allow ourselves to feel deep love and compassion for our body and our soul, we make healthier choices. Treating ourselves unlovingly welcomes others to do the same. Loving yourself includes how you treat and talk to your body, the types of people you spend time with, and the behaviors you tolerate in relationships or at work. When you allow someone to take advantage of you, you are showing that you are not worthy of respect. It's a hard reality to learn, but people will go as far as they can when it comes to what someone will tolerate. If your boss knows you will work constantly or in a poor environment, then nothing will change. We can't expect others to treat us well when we are unkind to ourselves. You are responsible for voicing your needs in the workplace, in relationships, and in life. I have a difficult time standing up for myself; I consider the other person's feelings more than my own. I've learned that standing up for myself is not mean or selfish but a way to show that I matter and that I will always take care of myself. We are all worth it. Don't be afraid to fight for yourself out of fear that you are asking for too much. Having your own back is a wonderful demonstration of how much you love yourself, and you are the most important recipient of this love.

DAY 320

Heartbreak, loss, endings, and tragedies all bring with them a certain amount of wreckage. Unwanted life events force parts of us to the surface or break open parts that once were intact. The heart is somewhat simple to use as an example, but the heart is also our greatest touch point to our experience. We "feel" things in our heart, joys and sorrows alike, but what is this part of us that feels heartache? How can an organ physically ache with no sign on a medical exam and no proof that anything is wrong? A broken heart is basically undetected—except by the person going through it— but that doesn't make the experience any less real. A broken heart feels tender, constricted, and painful.

It's fine to say our heart is broken; we are experiencing a lost person, relationship, or time in our life. Endings bring grief, and this often means a tender, "broken" heart. We think of a broken heart as needing time to heal; we tell ourselves it won't always be this way. What we might not realize is that when we endure loss or heartbreak, something new takes root. This could be a bad habit or addiction as an unhealthy way to cope. We can also grow from our experience, feeling our way through the pain and tenderness and acknowledging the uncomfortable sensations. When healing is continuous, it is a journey into new awareness. We arrive a new person with a deeper, more accurate identification of what it means to love. Maybe our heart was never meant to stay intact. Maybe we are here to feel, love, and grieve so we can experience the truth of our heart's capacity.

DAY 321

I was nine, sitting on the hill across from my grandmother's house. Shiny buttercups and puffy dandelions dotted the entire landscape, making the green grass all but disappear. I discovered a white daisy, plucked its straight stem, and examined the silky petals. One by one, I began pulling the petals and reciting, "*He loves me, he loves me not, he loves me, he loves me not, he loves me …*" As I lifted each petal from its root, my heart filled with anticipation of love and the promise that love would save me.

Like the childhood game teaches, I thought my experience of love was tied to another person and my worthiness of love was based on how someone else felt about me. We expect another person's love to save us. We believe another person's love somehow has a role in whether or not we actually love and accept ourselves. Our selfish viewpoint of love comes from long-held beliefs like the silly flower game. *I will be complete when he loves me.* Love is an offering and a practice. Love is something we are, not something we are owed.

I think about my grandma's hill, the flowers, and my desire for love, and I wish the game would have gone like this, "*I am love, I am love, I am love …*" What a world it would be if we knew we already are love and that we don't need to rely on another person to experience it. What a world it would be if we acted in love 100 percent of the time and trusted that—even when we're in the darkest places—love is still with us, holding us and keeping us safe, saving us and reminding us we already are.

DAY 322

The path of love is to remember your own capacity for unconditional love—as the giver and the receiver—regardless of other people. I cannot say if my heart aches more from being loved or being hurt; they are eerily similar. Moments that allow us to feel our own heart bring us more in tune with love. During yoga, during meditation, or even during a drive in the car when a particular cloud passes by, I feel held, and I understand love. The feeling is not like a movie or a fairy tale but a palpable awareness of oneness, of connection, and of something everlasting that will never go away. I glimpse that love is always available to me, no matter what is happening in my outside world, and I am able to return to this feeling of love simply by shifting my gaze to my own heart space and asking, *"What do you need today? What does my heart ache to tell me?"*

I admit, loving oneself feels a bit embarrassing, but try it. Try saying "I love you" to yourself in the mirror, and do it without laughing. I say "I love you" to friends, family, and my dog, but I have trouble admitting the words to myself. If saying it is too much of a leap, then try "I'm sorry," and "I'm sorry I have never checked in with you." Say these words to yourself, and when you feel your heart expand in your chest and become tender, when you feel the grief of having turned away from yourself, when you comprehend that you've had this power all along, watch your heart thump loudly and excitedly, as if saying, *"I've been waiting for you."*

DAY 323

My heart has spoken to me my entire life as my guide, my cheerleader, and my anchor, but through the busyness of the day-to-day, it's hard to make space to actually listen.

I spent two days in complete silence while at my yoga teacher training. I locked up my phone, so I had no access to calls, texts, or social media. After yoga all day, some walking, and silent eating in the dining hall, I found myself a little bored and slightly anxious. I sat in a comfortable chair and tried to meditate, and it was as if my heart had been waiting for this moment for me to really get quiet. I had nowhere to run. The opening of silence made space for some junk to float up from the depths. I took out my journal and wrote. There was no one to call and no other distraction. I wrote about past pain and experiences, and I was surprised at how many pages flowed out. Truthfully, I have never even read these pages. In the moment, I wrote to a scared little girl who needed to be held. I wrote to a confused woman who needed to know her strength.

My heart had been waiting a lifetime for me to notice these feelings. Maybe that's where my fear of abandonment comes from. Maybe it's not fear of a person leaving me but fear of me never returning to myself. Stay with your heart instead of trying to stay busy or reason your way out. Everything else will still be there, and acknowledging your heart is the greatest gift you can offer yourself.

DAY 324

Do you remember what it feels like to be in love? Not the circumstance or the events but the actual feeling in your body?

Hearing my baby cry in the middle of the night, I groggily walk down the hall to the nursery and click on the small table lamp so I can see. The baby stops crying as soon as I place my hand on his fluttering chest and scoop him up cozily with my other arm. Despite my crippling sleep deprivation, sore breasts, and aching body, I feel all wrapped up in peace and love.

Sitting beside my grandmother, knowing it would be the last time I saw her or looked into her eyes, I squeezed her hand and tried to decide on the best final words. I spoke, but my throat caught, and I said, "Don't worry. I'll see you soon." So strange. These are the last words I said to her. I don't even know if they were right. When I think of her, I remember her eyes, her skin on my hand, and I feel completely loved.

I believe that love is accessible in the darkest circumstance and that love truly never dies. The memory of something as powerful and present as love stays with us—in our body and in our being. The love in our heart cannot be destroyed or snuffed out unless we allow it. By turning our gaze toward love, by recalling a person who invokes this feeling, love becomes reality. We are right there, in the presence of our beloved, and nothing can take that away.

DAY 325

"I'm sorry," he said. "This is all on me."

My insides squirmed a bit but then let go. I responded, "Thank you." Raindrops sprinkled onto the windows and matted down the freshly cut grass. I had just mowed the lawn the day before, the second time since he moved out. My ex-husband apologized. I wasn't perfect either. I broke vows in different ways.

While married, we each settled into roles we never discussed or asked for. He mowed the lawn, and I mopped the floors. He paid the bills, and I bought diapers. We operated this way for years, never questioning our roles or where they came from. Now that I'm single, the old chores, such as cutting the grass and changing light bulbs, have become my rights of passage. They've become mundane, daily reminders that I am capable of more than I gave myself credit for. Likewise, the domestic tasks that used to define me no longer hold the same weight or smell of the same resentment. Every sacred object has been placed on the chopping block for final judgment—the wine glass, the strewn-about toys, the gnarly bushes by the front door. *Does this matter to me? At what cost?* Maybe we all need an honest self-assessment followed by a subtle rearranging of our roles, a conversation that shakes us awake and opens our eyes to the absurdity of our small life. Maybe we dig in—deep—and instead of arguing about details of the home or who is pulling their weight, we say what we actually feel, even though it risks us having to say the hardest things ever when felt from the heart: *"I'm sorry,"* and *"Thank you."*

DAY 326

Practicing love means finding balance with our responsibilities and knowing how to disperse our energy. Our energy is essential to our well-being. It's important to have enough self-awareness to know when we are sending too much energy out and not keeping enough for ourselves. And it's not the same from one day to the next. At times, we may be able to give everything; other times, we may need more self-care than usual. One way we act violently toward ourselves is by not listening to our energy and neglecting ourselves for the sake of projects or others.

Luckily, restoring our energy is pretty simple and fast. When life gets too full of "doing," make time to just be. Being restores our energy. Being supports our needs and desires. Make self-love and self-care a priority so you can enjoy all the activities and people you love. Commit to a few minutes of meditation, prepare a healthy meal, or say no to certain obligations. You'll find that after five minutes of quiet attention on yourself, you can give more and be more effective.

I know when I have few resources left because I get crabby, tired, impatient, and forgetful. Self-care and self-acknowledgment are beautiful practices because they allow us to show up in life as our best Self. We have so much to give. Our energy has the capacity to expand far and wide, reaching those we interact with and those we don't even know. When we take the time to cultivate our own "being," we are able to enjoy and support all the people and wonders of life.

DAY 327

Do something brave. By stepping out of your comport zone and not playing small, you show how much you love yourself. You have a right to your biggest dreams, and you are always protected. When you don't play life safe, you learn a lot about how you treat yourself during times of fear or inadequacy. Notice when you do something brave (or *think* about doing something brave). What thoughts come up? They may be fearful thoughts about why you shouldn't do it, why you can't handle it, or how you will fail. We try to talk ourselves out of something before we even try! This is an opportunity to quiet your critical voice, trust your heart, and move through the fear. Sometimes, we believe in the myth that pursuing dreams is selfish, but it's the opposite. Going after dreams honors our truth and demonstrates our worthiness. Going after dreams means you love yourself. Doing something brave might be telling someone how you feel or taking a risk in a relationship. It might be putting yourself out there. When the fear arrives, lean into your intuition instead of being pulled by your chattering mind. You never know how things will turn out. People may surprise you. The Universe may surprise you. We are here to be delighted and overcome with the love that is in store for us. If at first it appears that speaking your truth or going after something worthwhile makes opportunities or people fall away, know that this is also the Universe working in your favor. Those things weren't meant for you or in your best interest, but the surprise is still on its way. It is never wrong to follow your heart.

DAY 328

Be careful giving advice, even when it feels like the loving thing to do. We have no idea of someone else's experience and therefore no idea of their journey or their path. Listening provides an opportunity for someone to share, without our advice or critique. Unknowingly, we can impose violence on others when we tell them what to do or when we think we know what's best for them. It is wonderful to support and love others through their struggles, but when we try to fix them or change their path, we actually rob them of their growth. We can try to help too much, and we need to check our motives. Have faith that others are able to handle pain and discomfort—just like we are learning to handle our own challenges. Telling someone the solutions to their problems—trying to do the work for them— assumes their suffering has no merit and no purpose. All discomfort leads to growth, but we need to be the one to get ourselves there. Listening without responding or reacting is a difficult yet compassionate way to hear someone. We all have the capacity to figure our lessons out and to make changes when we've had enough, but we are the only ones who can determine when we are ready. Not only are we all capable of the same growth but we are all responsible. There is no benefit in stealing someone's insight by doing it for them or assuming we know the path that is best for them. Holding them in loving space by listening honors their journey and supports them more than you know.

DAY 329

Act as if you have no history, no experience, and no person who told you who to be. Act as if you are complete just as you are right now. Act from a place of beginning instead of looking back. We depend on others to tell us who we are, especially if we are abused, oppressed, or in the minority. When we step into our own person, both personally and politically, we give less power to those who told us who to be, and we destroy the assumption that we needed them to form our identity. Someone told you you were ugly, and you believed them. Someone told you you were worthless, and you believed them. Someone told you you would never get by without them, and you think this is the truth. It's interesting to notice how many things or people we allow to dictate our identity and form our choices. Consider this: If you are none of the things you've been told—if you are already worthy, beautiful, and capable—what would no longer matter? Would your choices change? Would your motives change? Would your wants change? How will you move forward? It's time to bravely step into that person and be free from the bonds of the past.

DAY 330

We can mistake self-compassion for self-care. However, a self-care routine does not necessarily mean we are treating ourselves kindly and with compassion. A self-care routine can be done out of retaliation, out of judgment, out of self-loathing, or out of criticism. So, it's important to acknowledge the intention behind our behaviors and listen to the ways we talk to ourselves.

I've noticed that it's easy for me to get mad at myself after a mistake and hard to let it go. I've noticed it's challenging not to self-criticize when I fall out of routine or balance. I've noticed that when I doubt my own capacity, I take it out on others by trying to make myself feel superior. Exploring unconditional love has made me realize that deep down I *want* to be perfect. But that's not where any of the lessons, wisdom, or *love* exists. It's true love when you love every single part of a person. Without moments of imperfection, we'd never have the chance for unconditional love. We'd never have the chance for forgiveness. We'd never have the chance to put compassion—for ourselves and others—into practice.

Instead of engaging in your self-care routine from a place of trying to prove something or from a place of lack, try adding self-compassion. Instead of thinking, "*I will be worthy when …,*" know you are already worthy. You are already beautiful. You are already strong. Your practice brings what is already within you out. We can always improve and reach for more, but we want to treat ourselves kindly along the way and come from a place of knowing our self-worth instead of punishing ourselves for not being better.

DAY 331

Everyone has their reasons for their actions and beliefs. Whether someone is aware or not, their entire existence is dependent on their experience. No one needs to know "why" they think and do things, but there's always a reason. Everyone's reactions to life are different. Two people can have the exact same experience and move through the aftermath in very different ways. And I believe no way is wrong or better. The biggest factor to whether or not someone is in pain is if they feel they are. We don't need to justify someone else's right to pain. We don't need to search for silver linings or point out how things could be worse. Just like we know how to feel our pain in order to help it move, we can sit next to others in their pain. We support their pain rather than try to change their experience. This is empathy; it is accepting someone's pain as it is. We carry all kinds of pain from the past into present experience. To accept someone's pain is to acknowledge their experience, which we know nothing about. We cannot travel into someone's pain. We cannot live where they have lived. The only way to touch someone's pain is to live through a similar experience and get a glimpse of the sensations and emotions firsthand. Even then, our picture of pain is based on our experience, not theirs. Listening without assumption or judgment provides the greatest insight into where someone has been and what they are going through.

DAY 332

If we knew the amount we were loved, regardless of rejection or others' behaviors, we would make very different decisions. We would be less afraid of acting a certain way and more able to act according to who we are, knowing that we are loved anyway.

When someone treats us unlovingly, we understandably take it personally, but often the amount of hurt we experience has more to do with feeling unloved than it does with the action itself. So, what if we knew we were loved anyway? What if we saw another's bad behavior as completely separate from our own worthiness of love? Would we respond differently? If we are betrayed or hurt by those we love, we immediately attribute their behavior to our own shortcomings. We can even blame ourselves and think that if we weren't the way we are, this never would have happened to us. Truthfully, the actions of others have little to do with us and much to do with the other person; they have to do with where they are human and where they are hurting. To not be affected is unreasonable, but to further treat yourself unlovingly is within your control. The actions of others never define you. There is no justification for being lied to, abused, or betrayed. To recognize someone's mistake and acknowledge the hurt it caused while also knowing you didn't deserve it is to walk the path of love with all its complexities. When you've been hurt, love yourself more. When you've been hurt, see the humanness in others. Continue to love because it is the only way through a broken, healing heart.

DAY 333

I believe that everyone has the same capacity to love. Some choose the path of love, and some don't. We have no true idea about anyone's experience except our own. Even when we share a similar experience with someone, it's impossible to understand the precise effects and what that person's inner landscape feels like.

We cannot control other people or outcomes, but we can change ourselves. We can lead by example. Yoga is not a self-fulfilling practice. Yoga is a practice in being a source of love. Love is so simple yet impossible to put into practice at times. Before I get to love, I must often arrive at denial, judgment, blame, and self-righteousness.

The good news is that all of our practices have been teaching us and bringing us the experience of love. Swami Kripalu describes our practice as three streams: devotion, knowledge, and yoga. He calls these "different wrappings for the same underlying experience, which is love."[66] You've been practicing and learning about love this entire time. The practice of love is arriving wide open in the field of surrender. The practice of love is remembering what we can and cannot control. The practice of love is being humbled into not having a solution and encouraged to enact faith. What would it look like to act as a source of love in this moment? What would you do to access that indestructible part within you? Knowing love is the source and the steadfast truth, what does love look like for you today?

....
66. Levitt, *Pilgrim of Love*, 141.

PRACTICE 12
Transformation (Dharma)

Dharma is our soul's path and our sacred duty. We all have a purpose on this earth. You might even get hung up on the question "What is my purpose?" Your purpose cannot be figured out with your mind; your purpose erupts from deep within you, and it is guided by your heart as well as the Universe. Your purpose is your essence, and your role is to keep searching in order to bring it out. There are many ways to discover our dharma, which I will share in the following readings. However, to find our purpose, we can observe what is happening right now. Our current experience is also our path and our purpose. Dharma is not outwardly famous, but everyone's dharma is extraordinary. By bravely and faithfully walking the path that is meant for us, by seeing our dharma through, we are fulfilled and content. We also serve the greater good. *Dharma* means "transformation" because the path changes us and everyone around us.

DAY 334

Dharma is called our sacred duty. Dharma is sacred because following our dharma connects us to our higher Self, our inner calling. Dharma is duty because as we seek out our dharma, we also serve others. You might not think your journey is meaningful enough to help another person, but everything you have been through and everything you have overcome, someone else is just beginning. Knowing that we help and serve others as a result of our experience makes even painful journeys worthwhile. Our path and our healing will help others heal.

Dharma can be a career, family, hobby, passion, or combination. Dharma is yours, and it doesn't have to look like anyone else's. Dharma is a path and not a destination. Along the path, we transform. What has transformed you? Dharma comes from your heart's longing. What interests you? What did you seek out as a child? What books do you like, and whom do you admire? These are all clues to your own unique dharma. Dharma is not easy or linear. We learn from our path, which is meant to be bumpy and unsure. Even when we are following our dharma, we may question it along the way. It won't always feel "good" or "right." But a part of you will know if you should keep going. With awareness and compassion, as we have been practicing all year, you can trust when your heart tells you to keep going. Deep down, you know if you are being truthful about where you are and what you want. Continue to move toward what lights you up. Don't settle and don't compromise. All dharma paths are meaningful, and all are sacred.

DAY 335

Another quality of dharma is that we live our own truth instead of someone else's. This means creating the life we want instead of the life someone else wants for us, but more than that, it means living according to our own values—as well as our definition of success. We live in a society that values money and material possessions. Despite society's prodding to accumulate fame, notoriety, and wealth, material gain has proven over and over to not be an absolute road to happiness. Fame may be someone's dharma but possibly not yours. It's an easy answer to say we all value money. And yes, money is necessary, but the idea that we will not be happy without a huge amount of money or that the way to achieve happiness is through something material is so ingrained from birth, it's almost impossible to consider that we may not be fulfilled this way. *What lights you up?* Is it getting a big paycheck, or is it the way your job of helping people makes you feel? Is it spending time with children? Is it a creative pursuit? Where do you actually find value, regardless of society's definition? The path to happiness is through our own fulfillment, not someone else's dharma or what fulfills them. We are not all fulfilled the same way, and that's what's so beautiful and amazing. You might be fulfilled through watching plants grow, inspiring people with your poetry, or building architecture. You are fulfilled by the action, by the doing, by the bringing forth of your own unique truth. When we try to live according to someone else's values, it's easy to get very muddy about our own.

DAY 336

If the idea of your soul's purpose scares you, good. It's pretty big. The first time I heard about dharma, I was so excited to find mine. *Yay! I have a calling! What is it? Is it grand? Is it exhilarating? Will it help people?*

Dharma is all of these things—grand, exhilarating, and of service. Dharma is essential to the greater good. Dharma has some qualities that are helpful as we consider our calling. First, dharma points to your inner essence. Dharma is about bringing forth what is within you, regardless of an exterior view. Building on that, dharma has little to do with outside success; dharma doesn't promise fame or fortune. Dharma has to do with how you feel. Lastly, the path to discovering your dharma will transform you. You'll gain wisdom and lessons.

To dive in a little more, here are some journal prompts:

+ What were you interested in as a child? What were your natural desires, and where did the world lead you?
+ Who are your heroes and mentors? Whom do you admire? Whom do you look up to?
+ What activities make time stand still? When do you feel fully at peace and almost meditative? What are you doing when you feel fully alive and present with the activity?
+ Where has there been synchronicity in your life? Consider jobs you've had or directions that arrived in an unexpected way. Where have opportunities shown up for you that you never would have thought of on your own? These synchronies can be the Universe showing you your dharma.

DAY 337

To "know thyself," as Plato says, is the one thing we can do in this lifetime to free ourselves from every single crutch, painful story, bad habit, and unhealthy cycle. The problem is that to know thyself is not so simple. It might take an entire lifetime just to figure out, and even if we do know ourselves, we might be too afraid to ever reveal who that person is. We might even be in denial.

Children seem to know themselves more easily than adults. Or maybe they just feel more permission to express whatever comes up and out of their bodies. But pretty quickly in life, children seek approval from parents, caregivers, teachers, and friends, and they slowly learn to add layers that cover up their true essence. Recovering our true Self might look like recovering from an illness, an addiction, or a relationship. Something shakes us awake in life, and we realize we are no longer okay hiding our true Self. When we see our current circumstance as the path, then everything we do to *recover* ourselves becomes our dharma.

The world can handle who you really are. We're so afraid to show up as ourselves we even lie to our *own Self* about who we are and what we want. It's the biggest travesty in existence because every one of us has something to give to this world, to our children, to our jobs, and to our partners just exactly as we are. Not when we learn the new *thing*, get the degree, lose the weight, or heal past the *whatever*— but right now, walking our current path and living our purpose.

DAY 338

Your dharma will continue to show you lessons. So, while dharma is exhilarating and liberating, dharma is also challenging and possibly painful. Lessons we thought we had dealt with may resurface from time to time, signaling there is more work to do. Even once we decide to let a limiting belief go, it can creep back into our experience. It's exhausting. I know the frustration of trying desperately to be rid of something, especially when I am logically aware of how ridiculous it is, only to be continually reminded that it is still part of me.

Don't be deceived. If you are on a journey to uncover your pain, if you are actively seeking a new lifestyle, a new perspective, or a new way of talking to yourself, the journey will look a lot like falling down at first. The journey will look like you can't get it right—until you do. Removing layers of self-doubt, self-criticism, and self-hatred takes a lot of practice. Beliefs have been with us for a lifetime, and chances are they have found their way into everything we do. Even when we heal one layer, there are more layers underneath. *How deep do you want to go? How free do you want to be?* To be on the path of transformation is to always be learning, rising, falling, and rising again. There is no end other than fulfilling our purpose along the way. You're not doing anything wrong if something is presenting itself again. This is another growth point and another opportunity for transformation. You know exactly what to do because you have been here before. This is bringing you to the next level.

DAY 339

I believe that your desires are not an accident. Your desires are within you because they are possible. Nothing is out of reach. Nothing is "too much." Your inner desires point to what will fulfill you and what will benefit the world. Unfortunately, we may have been conditioned to think that our desires are frivolous or selfish and that acting on an inner calling is impractical at best. We've bought into the myth that we shouldn't aim to feel fulfilled every day, that this isn't even realistic. We accept that we may not be able to answer our true calling in our daily life or work. But what if our life was our calling? Part of the practice of yoga is to discover our calling and go after it.

Our calling connects us to our true Self and to the greater energy outside us. Yoga aims to liberate us from human suffering by awakening our soul, and this happens when we pursue our dharma at all costs. Our calling is precisely why we are here, and by ignoring it, we are not only preventing ourselves from being fulfilled, but we are also dismissing the greater plan. To do the inner work it takes to know our calling—and to have the courage to bring it forth—aligns us with the Divine. To go after our calling is to live a spiritual life; by living a spiritual life, we are fulfilled.

This concept of dharma brings up so many questions. Can a calling be simple? Mundane? Does the mail carrier have a calling, and is it delivering the mail? Yes, it can be. Dharma is not about the external; it is about that which is awakened within you. Yes, it is possible to feel fulfilled every single day of your life.

DAY 340

All you have to do is stay on the path. Once you know you have an essential purpose and that this gift already exists within you, your entire life becomes part of your dharma. Your path does not have to be figured out from the start, like choosing what you want to be when you grow up, deciding where to go to school, and what to study. Your path can be wandering and full of detours; your path is not direct but seeking and staying open. Even before we know anything about dharma, we are already on the path. But when we do know—when we start paying attention—life gets really exciting. Notice when synchronies arrive, and you will sense they are signs pointing you a certain way or telling you, *"Yes! This is right. Go here!"*

All of it is your dharma. You don't have to try so hard to figure it out. When you do something that fulfills you, you'll know it, and you'll keep doing it. That one miraculous moment, when you choose to honor yourself and keep doing that which fulfills you, is momentous. Too often we dismiss what erupts from within. Too often we think we are crazy. We call our longings silly or pointless. Write, if you are called to write. You don't need a plan; just do the action of bringing the thing forth. Play an instrument, join a club, cook a favorite recipe, keep seeking, and keep going. If you're paying attention, all your choices that answer the internal nudges from your soul will lead you straight (or winding) to your dharma. There is no other way.

DAY 341

I never expected my recovery to become a spiritual path. I just wanted to quit drinking because it was causing so many problems in my life. But then recovery became many things. It wasn't just quitting booze but also practicing meditation and yoga, attending therapy, addressing disordered eating, addressing codependency, feeling my emotions, and being present. When I tore off the alcohol Band-Aid, I opened up a slew of self-violating patterns I had been practicing my entire life.

Like recovery, I never expected yoga to become a spiritual path. Yoga started as a way to get out of my house. Yoga started as an escape. But once there, on my mat, I observed sensations in my body, and instead of running from them or drowning them with wine, I stayed. I cried on my mat, and I let my heart break wide open in camel pose. Without my addiction, without my yoga mat to feel, without everything that got me to this point, I never would have started taking care of myself. I never would have known I could change. I never would have stood up for myself, fought for myself, or loved myself. I never would have pursued my writing.

Before life fell apart, I was going through the motions because that was what I had been conditioned to do—ignore problems and be happy. Get a good job and be grateful. By turning toward my problems, my supposed failures, and my messes, I allowed spirit to step in.

Stop asking, *"Why me?"* Instead, try to ask, *"What is this here to teach me?"* When you allow an experience to transform you, it is dharma.

DAY 342

In my dream, I was riding my bike downhill. The front tire was flat and stuck in a deep and muddy rut. Despite being on an incline, I stood still. I kept putting my foot down to push, but I couldn't get out of the sunken groove.

I always want to get places faster than is reasonable. I want to get *through* something in order to be somewhere else. I can see the bright and shiny light dancing at the end of the tunnel, and it all but blinds me. The end is so distracting and inviting that I forget about all the work that needs to be done to get there.

When we have a big project at hand, a goal to achieve, or a life stage to "get through," it's important to remember that the process of getting there is so much more rewarding than our image at the end. The tunnel is your teacher and your safe place. The tunnel is what you will remember; it's the part that will stay with you because it reminds you of who you really are. The tunnel is your calling.

When the tunnel is dark and there seems to be no light at the end, stay. Dark times are when we recognize that we actually have light inside us. When you are happy, you might think external sources are providing your light—the relationship, the job, the perfect body, the perceived success—but it is none of these things. It is you. You are the light you seek. When you're stuck in the tunnel, you're not really stuck. You're being asked to stay because magic is happening there, and you don't want to miss it.

DAY 343

I always remind students in a balance pose that it makes no difference if you stay balanced the entire time or if you fall out and come back. It makes no difference if you use a wall or a prop. Holding the pose versus tipping and returning has no effect on the benefits or the results. Even when you fall, your muscles are still learning. Your core is still toning. In fact, in the coming back, your body is getting stronger. The same applies to your mind. When the mind gets critical or off topic, bring it back. Holding a tranquil mind for long periods of time has little added benefit compared to when we continually bring the mind back; both scenarios are training the mind. Both are how the Bhagavad Gita describes yoga as "skill in action."[67]

In life, don't get disturbed by things not going your way or as expected. Your reaction to outside circumstance or supposed setbacks does not have to be one of disappointment or failure. If you are engaged in the action, do so fully, without ties to outcome or appearance. When we are devoted to and fully present in action, the results do not matter. The messiness along the way also does not matter. Journeys that are perfect do not lead you somewhere better than journeys that are difficult. Why do we expect the journey to be easy and without falls? Yoga teaches us to be fully committed to our practice and our pursuits; this focus on the action, rather than the result, will deliver us the fruits that are meant for us.

....
67. Easwaran, *The Bhagavad Gita*, 94–95.

DAY 344

Look around. See your life as it is in all its glory, joys, mistakes, trials, and successes. Our beliefs are powerful. Our beliefs affect our perceptions and, therefore, our actions. What have you been telling the Universe? Energy attracts a similar vibration. This is why people often experience a bad day getting worse. The morning starts with spilled coffee and a traffic jam, and throughout the day, there are numerous accidents, trip-ups, or delays. On these days, we wonder why we ever got out of bed. Our energy started out low. Maybe we were tired and clumsy. We stayed down in that wallowing energy, and our day never recovered. Likewise, when our vibration is high, like the energy of love, joy, service, or gratitude, we attract more of that. We've all experienced moments, days, or weeks when everything seemed to just flow. That's not an accident; that's energy.

The mind is an excellent teacher. When we observe the mind, we gain insight into the messages we may be sending to the Universe. We gain awareness of our thoughts and beliefs. In order for the Universe to respond to what we want, we need to be focused and forthright. We need to know we deserve what we are asking for and move forward with action. If you say to the Universe, "I want to be a published author," but never write a page, you have just confused the Universe. We are in constant communication with the Universe. Let your actions demonstrate your intention. Take heart that the action is your part, and the rest is up to the loving energy that surrounds you.

DAY 345

Sometimes, I imagine I am living several different lives at once, all a result of different choices, circumstances, and decisions. Had I gone there, chosen this, not been so full of self-doubt, then where would I be? *If I knew then what I know now...*

We wouldn't know what we do today unless everything that happened yesterday happened. We are not the same person today as we were yesterday or five years ago, so it is impossible to expect that person from our past to have made any different choices than they did. But today is a new day; we can take the knowledge we have now and start today. We don't need to keep the past alive by continuing to make the same mistakes. We don't need to feed the same fears. It's never too late.

Where you are today is a result of everything you have experienced and everything you have overcome. Those lessons are priceless; use them from here on out. When we stop repeating the same behaviors from the past, we arrive in a new place. This is why we went through everything we did—to learn a new way. There is no need to regret or wallow in decisions from the past. In fact, you can flip your entire perspective and actually be grateful for every horrible, messy, or shameful wrong turn.

Your experience and all the events and choices that happened before this had a monumental impact on who you are today. Today, is 100 percent possible because of everything that came before. Starting from today, at this moment, make the most of it.

DAY 346

When we start changing and growing, some people fall away. Making healthy choices or choices that are best for you now doesn't sit well with everyone, but it doesn't matter what anyone else thinks. What matters is that you don't experience that sinking feeling anymore—that feeling of going against yourself in order to keep the peace. We fear the consequence of others' responses more than we fear the burden of staying small. Staying small means we refuse to advocate for ourselves. We refuse *our Self* in order to keep others comfortable. If you've spent much of your life making others comfortable, like I have, it can feel discouraging when you begin to set boundaries. All of a sudden, all the people you kept happy for so long retaliate. They express disappointment or get angry. They might try to change your mind.

If they do, stand strong. This is not the time to acquiesce or give up on yourself. You've set a magnificent course in motion, and it's important you see it through. That voice inside you is real. Your gut is real. You know when you're being called to answer it, even if the answer will make others upset.

Your life can look like whatever you want it to if you have the courage and the self-love to pursue it. Happiness and fulfillment come from within, not from anything external, which means the outside can look amazing and we can feel miserable. Likewise, the outside can look miserable to someone else and we can feel amazing. Trust your heart instead of others' opinions. It's hard to disappoint those we love, but they will come around. Inner peace and contentment are contagious.

DAY 347

The path of transformation is one of continually looking toward ourselves and our actions. Transformation is not an outer journey; it is not reaching for an end goal or prize. Transformation is an inward journey, one that slowly uncovers truth after truth.

Maybe all this running toward outside pleasure and satisfaction has been a tireless effort to escape ourselves. What if we placed as much or more merit on the inner journeys as we do the outer successes? Every time you look within, every time you discover a nugget of wisdom about how you act and why, you have just traveled a little further on your journey. Celebrate. Celebrate every moment you are brave enough to listen and learn something new. Even as you reach for your dreams, even as you seek out your dharma, do not minimize the lessons along the way. To practice yoga and focus only on achieving the pose is missing all the wisdom in the getting there—the doubt, the putting off, the critical voice, the staying, the resilience, and the victory. As we go, we might feel discouraged when there is always something to uncover and always something new to learn. The path is never ending. To be finished would be to die. Embrace each uncovering like a trophy. *Ah ha! Another lesson!* You are still here—growing, transforming, and never stagnant.

DAY 348

As long as there are new challenges, new fears, and new unknowns to explore, you are growing. Moving forward despite discomfort or fear takes a great amount of trust. Seeing other people put themselves out there reminds us what is possible. A few people I know personally are being brave every single day. One is stumbling through new sobriety but getting up each time, enacting the faith to try again. One is being vulnerable with a new partner, even though every cell in her body is reminding her what has happened in the past. One is helping a friend through the grief of her dad's death, even though it is triggering the loss of her own father. One is recognizing a long overdue conversation she needs to have with her mother.

Our bravery inspires others to be brave, and we heal each other along the way. Our past has the power to shut us down from love, from ourselves, and from life. The only way to reshape the past is to enter situations that may trigger us and notice how we react. If we can move through the trigger, if we can witness our past pain emerge and be able to hold it despite the discomfort, we can create a new future. The risk is worth it. We will not break open to the point of no return. These past scars are begging to be healed, and doing so requires a brave, open heart. "Baby steps," my mother-in-law used to say. Start small and observe others around you who are also being brave. Let their vulnerability inspire and support you. Today, right now, also acknowledge all the ways you are brave.

DAY 349
Future Self Meditation

Get comfortable. Take a few breaths and close the eyes. Observe the breath for several rounds: inhale, exhale. With every breath, let the body become more relaxed. Imagine you are a child and go to a place from your childhood; it can be a real place or made up. Visualize the place in terms of all the sights, sounds, smells, and touches. You are your child Self. Next, imagine your future Self walking toward you. Let the image of your future Self be whatever comes to mind. Visualize how that person looks, what they are wearing, and how they approach you. Ask your future Self a question, or see if they have a message for you. If nothing comes, get a sense of the feeling they bring you. It could be bravery, love, or insight about a project. Spend some time as your child Self interacting with the energy of your future Self. Let your future Self guide the moment; you don't have to force anything. Be open and listen with your entire body.

Our future Self exists in energetic potential and is a version of us who is wiser and more knowing. When we bring ourselves back to childhood and meet our future Self during meditation, we are tuning in to the energy that is both the child and the wise Knower. Both versions of us exist today, and this meditation allows for conversation between the two in order to gain comfort, advice, or simply connection. Greet your future Self. Be open to the child as you learn from the wiser you. Often, we need support and direction when finding our way. Your future Self is a great resource; they are you.

DAY 350

We are always moving beyond different points of comfort in order to keep going and continue growing. We might settle into a familiar place or energy state, but as energy shifts and expands, so do we, and so does our experience. The minute you think you have the answer, you are stuck. We, of course, meet triumphs and insight along the way, but these moments of knowing lead us directly to the next question, the next unknown. Your entire journey, which probably started out as a way to seek answers, has now become a process in being comfortable with the fact that there is no answer, no guarantee. The answer is in the constant awareness of life's temporary nature and the shifting of experience. The minute you feel good and attach to the person or circumstance you believe is making you feel that way, something changes. The nature of the world shows you that, once again, there is no purpose in relying on the external to hold you up. We are not meant to attach to an outside source for our fulfillment. Through the temporality of life and because we cannot control the outside world, we are constantly reminded that fulfillment must come from within. Fulfillment does not mean happiness all the time. Answering and exploring the call from within takes discomfort, asking questions, observing, and moving through fears. Every edge we meet brings new lessons and new awareness. We learn to be less surprised by what arrives in a day or a year and more accustomed to the freedom of watching everything pass by. Movement becomes our nature, even though it brings changing emotions and experiences.

DAY 351

Name it. And then go after it with everything you have. It's possible you know exactly what you want. Even though we each have an innate gift, one that was handed to us from the heavens or beyond, we second-guess whether or not it is real. Should we bring it forth? What if it doesn't work out? For some reason, answering our calling brings up a lot of fear. We get so hung up on the details, we stop ourselves before we even get started. Your only task is to start. Once you start, the Universe will respond with the next move and the next. You don't have to have everything laid out in front of you or even an end in sight. We create so much drama and consternation by analyzing everything as we go. If we could just trust that in the big picture everything will work out, we'd avoid a lot of unpleasant feelings along the way. I have seen time and time again when someone begins going after their calling and the most surprising opportunities arrive. They usually end up in an entirely different place than they had planned but are still able to live out their calling. We don't need to cling to certain details of our dharma. In fact, this can prevent us from seeing the opportunities that are actually in store for us. If you're pursuing your calling and it appears to be at a dead end, stay open. Let go of the wheel for a bit, and ask yourself what this experience is telling you. Setbacks are not telling you to give up; they're opening space for what is meant to arrive.

DAY 352

Where is your focus and your energy? Is it aligned with the intentions of the Universe, or are you off trying to make your own things happen? I have spent hours, days, and years trying to orchestrate my life on my terms. If I could just step back and allow the Universe to guide me, I would feel much more at ease. We forget that we are not in charge. When it comes to dharma and our soul's path, we are always in collaboration with the Universe and the greater plan. Often, the things I am supposed to be doing for my own path and the greater good are the exact things I resist. This is not done intentionally, but I wander off to someone else's dharma, someone else's path, and try to make mine look like theirs. I believe I have found my way, and without asking my higher Self, I bulldoze ahead. I waste precious energy trying to be someone else, and I always fall short. Desperate, I come back to my heart and ask, *"What happened? Why didn't that work?"* As usual, I wasn't listening. I was letting my ego run the show instead of being open. I thought I knew the answer instead of being comfortable in the unknown. We are not in charge. If the Universe isn't responding to your manic efforts to make something happen, pay attention. Stop doing and get still. Where are you being led? Where does the Universe want (and need) your energy? Observe the actions that brought you here, and ask how you can be more open. Also ask yourself what has arrived without you forcing it? That's where you want to put your focus.

DAY 353

As soon as you understand that nothing outside of yourself will complete you, you have become free. I cannot say I have achieved this state, which Patanjali calls *dharmamegha* ("cloud of enlightenment"). After all, he describes it as a state when all desire is gone.[68] As we pursue our dharma, we do it from a place of present contentment and remain unattached to the outcome. I certainly don't know how to be human without desire or attachment, especially when I am going after my dharma—I want results.

I am comforted by the lessons from yoga, which remind me I can be aware of my desires while still practicing and seeking liberation. In this sense, yoga becomes a path of progress and constant exploration. We were not aware of our attachments before we started yoga. We just thought that was the way life was. Suddenly, when confronted with an attachment, we notice. We perk up and think, *"Oh yes! I am attached! Here is the lesson!"* Everything becomes an opportunity to practice, which frees us a little more and then a little more. Our awareness of the practice brings more peace, more contentment, less worry, and less desire. Events that used to derail us hold less power. We realize we are able to handle the uncertainty and the setbacks. We gain flexibility in body and in mind. We are not so easily pulled down into the depths when something goes wrong or we lose a little control. We observe the world happening around us and calmly remember, *"I never had control anyway."* It is magnificent.

....
68. Satchidananda, *The Yoga Sutras of Patanjali*, 214.

DAY 354

Freedom from desire and attachment is more attainable than you think. I am happy to point out and address some questions that are probably arriving and churning in your mind. If we are free from desire, then do we care about nothing? How do we go after our calling with full effort if we do not care? What is the point? Fulfilling your dharma is showing up, doing the effort full-out, and letting the outcome go. If you are in the middle of a fantastic project and all seems in flow with the Universe, but then you get sick, the sickness is now your dharma. Don't resist it. When I had kids, I tried to keep working as if nothing had changed. I was a new mom, but I clung to my old way of life, therefore missing the dharma of the moment. But should I do my dharma with no recognition? Don't I have to make a living? Yes, we all have responsibilities. We most likely can't run off to a mountain to write, sing, or paint. Yet somehow, when we start to own our gifts and our path, life shows up and reveals a new way. Your current job can support your lifestyle as well as your dharma. You can make sacrifices. You can take a class on evenings or weekends. An opportunity may present itself, and your dharma could become your income. Freedom from attachment is to remain open and teachable. Being free from desire doesn't mean we stop caring. It means we pay attention to what is in front of us, and rather than view it as an obstacle, we allow it to become part of our experience.

DAY 355

When someone rejects your dharma, either in conversation or blatant rejection, like when you're turned down for a job or get a "no" from an opportunity, it doesn't mean you have missed the mark. Rejection has nothing to do with your dharma. Remember, dharma is not about the external view but about your own internal fulfillment. If writing poetry fulfills you, if the act of putting down words and phrases brings you to a state of bliss and makes you feel more alive, this is your barometer, not what anyone else or the world thinks. Rejection and failure happen during any meaningful pursuit. We hear stories of famous athletes who never made the high school team and authors who were rejected numerous times before landing a book deal. The world is funny and surprising, and every rejection is a blessing in disguise. We either learn from it and keep going, or we give up and allow someone else to determine our fate.

In moments when we are at a loss, when we don't know the answer because we thought this was "it" and it just fell through, we arrive once again at surrender, the fifth of the five yamas in Patanjali's Sutras. Maybe we wallow for a bit and feel sorry for ourselves. We allow ourselves to consider giving up, even though we know we won't really. Like the dawn of a new day, we come back to our senses and back to our truth. *I must do this because it is who I am.* There is nothing braver, more freeing, or more in alignment with the Divine than being who you are and surrendering the entire path—triumphs and supposed tragedies—to something outside yourself.

DAY 356

Human beings want to feel purposeful. Through purpose, we are fulfilled. You'd think a person's sense of purpose—whether they are living a worthwhile existence—would be based on outside factors. Someone with a high-paying job and a "good" life feels fulfilled, while someone in a less desirable situation would find less purpose or meaning. However, this appears to not be the case. Someone living a "successful" life does not necessarily feel fulfilled, and someone living through a much more tragic situation is able to find deep meaning. Our sense of purpose comes from an inner knowing that life can change; we can change. No matter what your situation is today, something inside keeps you going. Maybe it's a hope for better days ahead or a project you want to see through. It's very common that between what is and what is yet to come, when we are on the brink of catapulting forward to our purpose, obstacles arrive, both internally and externally. You get ill. Your car breaks down. Someone needs you. Inside, you may feel agitated or doubtful. All of this tension, life's way of asking you if you're serious, is temporary. Something must be lost in order for something new to arrive. And we cling to the familiar, even if it's not what is best. Let go. Allow for any disturbances while staying rooted to your intention and your inner knowing. Let go and keep going.

DAY 357

When you are disturbed, sad, or stressed and you lend a hand to someone else, your act of kindness takes your own problems away. According to the Bhagavad Gita, being of service is one way to reach self-actualization and is therefore part of our yoga practice.[69] Listening to a friend or helping with a task has the power to take us out of ourselves. We remember our humanity and our connection; helping others lessens the weight of our own burdens. My struggle is that I never feel there is enough time. So, if I am already stressed about too much to do, the last thing I want is to add more to my plate by offering to help someone else. But when I remember, when I ask what I can offer—instead of what I want to receive—I immediately experience a shift in my perception. Most of our problems are, in fact, in our heads, or at least their severity is. We blow things out of proportion and want solutions *now*. Our problems, worries, and agitations do matter. However, we can prevent ourselves from spiraling into unnecessary self-wallowing when we make ourselves available for another human being. In my mind, I get nothing done; I only continue to feed the ego, and my tasks are very ineffective. Outside my mind, when focused on someone else, I release the pull of my own troubles and give myself a break. Afterward, a little lighter and fuller with love, I can accomplish much more and make healthier choices than had I stayed in my own drama. The person you helped will thank you, but actually, they helped you.

....

69. Easwaran, *The Bhagavad Gita*, 219.

DAY 358

You don't have to be good at your dharma, at least not right away. When I finally owned my dharma and really began to focus on daily writing in my late thirties, I thought I was brilliant. Feeling the joy writing brought me was like discovering a part of myself I never knew existed. I felt awake and alive, blissful. This was good—I kept writing. I felt like I had so much to say. Unlike when I spoke, the words seemed to flow out of me, filling the page. It almost seemed like someone else was writing for me, maybe my higher Self.

Today, when I read that writing from the first year, I wince. The writing is not good. It's clear I was writing for myself and not for anyone else. The way I improved my writing was by writing. Because I fell in love with the act of writing, I wrote every day, sometimes for hours and sometimes for minutes. I carried pads of paper with me to jot down ideas as they came, which was also an act of writing, observing my surroundings and experiences and putting them to words. I immersed myself in the writing process, and my *talent* improved the more I wrote. We think talent is innate, but our joy for the practice is what shapes our passions into talents. Our talents cannot be cultivated if we never engage in them. Fall in love with whatever it is that brings you bliss. Engage in your bliss daily. Don't let your mind tell you to stop because you are "no good." No one with any talent got there because they stopped practicing. Your heart has led you to this activity. Enjoy it, and your talent will grow from that joy.

DAY 359

Things falling apart and things falling into place look strangely similar. Certain beliefs, behaviors, and ways of life need to be undone or eliminated in order for new, more appropriate footing to arrive. If the ground is shifting beneath you, moving toward a new relationship, location, career, life stage, or goal, it might feel uneven, shaky, bumpy, or even painful at times. Trust that the earth will settle. Soon there will be solid ground and a new horizon. The shifting means change is happening. You are on a path, and there are no promises that it will be even.

During the settling, as we meet edges and learn new ways, it's tempting to backtrack. We remember our old life with a rosier, romanticized view, and if we glance in that direction, we wonder if we should return. Parts were good; parts are always good. But you started this journey for a reason—probably for many reasons. Remember them. Especially when fear arrives and you question where you are going, remember why you wanted this change. Your intuition was not a mistake. Your heart does not lead you astray. You've made it this far, and any churning from within is not a sign to turn back but an indicator of great change ahead.

When you arrive, you will know it. You will be able to breathe more deeply and look back on all the changes with gratitude and wonder. You will be able to stand on solid ground and understand you were guided the entire time.

DAY 360

True change and true growth look so natural it's hard to remember who you were before this transformation. When you embody the practices of yoga, the essence of who you are shifts from striving to welcoming, from complaining to being grateful, and from worrying to having absolute trust. Maybe some less desirable qualities are not completely gone from you, but notice how quickly you are able to spot them when they arrive. The practice becomes believing yourself. The practice becomes recognizing your center. The practice becomes smiling, laughing, letting go, tuning in, uncovering buried treasure, and owning your strength. Where you may have been afraid to look, you now crave this feeling of self-observation without judgment because you know every new awareness leads to more freedom. The practice becomes one of love, not only for yourself but for others, and the world appears less harsh without the lens of your own judgment and critique. Your body moves differently because it has changed. But beyond your physical form, you sense that something else is different. No one notices for a while, and then one day someone asks, "Is something different about you?" Just like people can spot pain and despair, they also recognize hope and appreciation. When people come in contact with someone who embodies love, confidence, or knowing, it's hard not to pay attention. The practice is contagious—and desirable. Maybe your outside world has changed: there is a new job, relationship, or adventure. But more than that, something inside of you has shifted. The gift of yoga is a shift in perception; where there was illusion, there is now truth.

DAY 361

The well-known image of Buddha finding enlightenment under the bodhi tree makes the idea of awakening seem like a solitary experience. Through yoga and meditation, we focus on drawing our attention inward to notice thoughts and sensations, to become increasingly aware of the emotional Self and the workings of the mind. Awakening is within you, so moments of enlightenment, of "pure awareness" like the yogis speak of, happen while we are alone and tuned in to our practice. But living a spiritual life and having an awareness of spirituality are two different things. Living a spiritual life by connecting with others is what keeps us on the path. There is little purpose in achieving enlightenment and keeping it all to yourself. To "walk the spiritual walk," we must not only become aware of our own capacity—as well as our own humaneness—but equally aware of those same qualities in others. Compassion, the ability to understand someone else as yourself, helps us experience love every day of our lives. We are connected not because we share the same beliefs, the same upbringings, or the same religion but because we share the same ability to be imperfect and continue seeking. My weakness helps me to recognize yours. My mistakes help me to forgive yours. My wounds help me to sit beside you with yours. My ability to fall and then rise helps me to know that you can do it too.

DAY 362

Despite teaching the transformational effects of yoga, it's still hard to believe the power of these practices—on myself and on my students. Do you believe it's all true? Have you seen your own transformation? We can live a life of boundless possibility and radical acceptance. We are powerful beyond our understanding. We are fiercely loved by something greater than we know. We are connected to every single human being on this planet—and maybe even to those who are no longer with us in physical form. Life is willing to delight us with people and situations beyond our imagination or what we would choose for ourselves. How did you get here?

You showed up. You trusted. You read these pages and became willing. You let yourself feel pain and pleasure without judgment. You glimpsed the possibility of trusting yourself. You accepted every good experience and bad experience as yours, and you held on to the idea that all of it was necessary. You began to test your own strength. You discovered you wouldn't die from feeling some discomfort or even pain. You took risks. You took rest. A year ago you were not the person standing here today. It's true for you and for everyone brave enough to go down this path of curiosity and self-reflection. Whatever brought you here, give it the appreciation it deserves. I believe that we are never in the wrong place at the wrong time, and every single moment is one of divine intervention. Maybe you feel you are not at an end but at a beginning; this means you have truly accepted your practice as one of lifelong learning, endless discovery, and infinite growth.

DAY 363

In seeking your dharma, do not mistake doing what fulfills you as making yourself happy all the time. The dharma path can be one of very uncomfortable emotions because transformation is just that—uncomfortable. If dharma transforms you, it points you straight toward everything you don't want to look at. If dharma wasn't your soul's purpose, it wouldn't require so much of your soul to go after it. Yoga postures teach us the difference between discomfort we can handle and pain. In a pose, we may have mistaken rising sensation as pain when really it was part of change. After a period of sustaining a pose, your muscles will feel on fire right before you come out. If you stay—when you stay—especially when the moment gets so intense you are about to jump off but instead you take one more breath, transformation happens. As you slowly bring your body out of the pose, as the burn subsides and you see the fruits of your effort, you know you are different.

It's the same with dharma. Right before the dream comes true, right before you get to the next summit, sensation will be intense. You've been climbing for a while with periods of excitement, periods of mild discomfort, and periods of pure bliss. At this point, you may be unprepared for the intensity that arrives right before the moment of transformation. There may be obstacles, emotions, and burning, much like the muscles during a pose that is about to bring change. Can you stay? Can you pay attention? Find or do one thing that will help you stay—maybe a word, a friend, a hand on your heart to remember who you are. Can you hold on for one more breath?

DAY 364
Walking Meditation

Find a spot where you can walk or take several steps. You can be inside or outside. Take off your shoes and socks. Once barefoot, stand for a moment on solid earth or floor. Notice what the surface feels like on the soles of your feet. Take an inhale and lift your heart space as if trying to connect with the sky. Rest your shoulders down, and let your arms hang at your sides. Feel the earth beneath your feet, wiggle into every sensation. Soft grass, muddy road, cement driveway, wooden floors, or smushy carpet. Your trusty mat. Only when you feel ready, lift one foot, and take a step. Savor that step, heel to toe. Then take the next step and the next. Walk slowly and mindfully around your space. Continue to breathe, offering your heart to the heavens each time.

Thank your feet for supporting you and for allowing these sensations. Thank your knees for bending and bruising. Thank your heart for being a safe hiding place and an offering. Walk mindfully as if this is the first time your feet have felt this surface. Maybe it is the first time, or at least the first time you've paid attention. Breathe deeply and fully, knowing your breath keeps you alive and brings you in touch with your soul. Breathe love and gratitude into each step, marveling at where you've been and where you are. Feel gratitude for this moment, gratitude for yourself, and gratitude for everything that has led you here.

DAY 365

I want you to know that at the beginning of writing this book—and maybe for you as you took on the task of reading it—365 days of spiritual teachings seemed a daunting undertaking. Doubt and fear swirled. How would I break it down? How long would it take? Is there enough to say? Anne Lamott's book *Bird by Bird* is a guide for writers and begins with a story about her dad helping her brother write a book report on birds. After having three months to complete the assignment, nothing is done, and the paper is due tomorrow. How do we accomplish the impossible? How do we get from *here* to *there* when "there" is so far away? As Lamott's dad says to her brother, "Bird by bird, buddy. Just take it bird by bird."[70] We create small, achievable tasks, and they add up to a whole new way of life. At the beginning, it seems messier than when we started. We ride the waves of doubt, excuse, and possibly even hatred. What starts off as deliberate self-discipline turns into our natural way of being. Day by day, our practice becomes who we are. Yoga is, all of a sudden, everywhere, and we see opportunities to practice in all our relationships and pursuits. This daily practice, this page-by-page journey that also invited you into action, is a testament to your ability to make the impossible possible and to arrive "here," which used to feel so out of reach. How did you do it? Was it love? Was it strength? Was it faith? It was all those things; it was also you. *You* got yourself here. Now, what else will you do?

....
70. Lamott, *Bird by Bird*, 19.

DAY 366

Happy Leap Year! An extra day, a bonus, and a blessing. What will you do with it? When I have extra time, I always try to fill it. I want to seize the opportunity and not waste it, but yoga teaches that we do not need to dive into an extra project or add more to our list in order to make the most of our time. This extra day is a wonderful opportunity to practice the third of the five yamas, *asteya*, which means nonstealing. Nonstealing refers to not taking physical things that are not ours, stealing the path or the successes of others, and not stealing time from our own experience. How do we steal our time? We get too busy. We rush through life without presence or mindfulness. We have little memory of where we have been because we were not paying attention while we were there. We were already on to the next thing. We leave no time to rest, reflect, or integrate our experience.

Here are some ideas to practice asteya today:

+ Pull out your journal from last year; flip through the pages and remember your experience, where you were, and where you are today.

+ Meditate for ten to twenty minutes and view all that has happened over the year, like a movie playing on a screen. Start at the beginning and take in the scenes. Notice what plays in your mind. Memories and moments might be big, mundane, and everything in between.

+ Rest. Take a nap or lie down in shavasana. Watch a movie. Go to bed early. Your body needs to integrate all the experiences of the year as well.

Conclusion

You have learned so much. If you've read this book—one page a day for an entire year—you've no doubt discovered new ways of seeing yourself and new ways of overcoming. Just like beginnings are exciting as well as scary because the path is unfamiliar and unknown, endings might also bring up a range of emotions and possibly a sense of grief. You may feel sadness for the ending or a wondering about what to do now. Whenever I finish a project or something that has required my effort and focus for a sustained period of time, there is a slight letdown at the end. I have been consumed, held, and immersed, and now I feel like I am being tossed out of the nest. You know what to do—notice it all.

Also know that your journey does not end here. These pages, words, and lessons are never ending and never fully absorbed. We are always facing new situations from a different sense of Self. Take some time to celebrate the last year and all you have accomplished. Then turn back to day 1 and begin again, or ask your soul to choose for you—flip to any page and read the practice. Every reading will be different. Something that was unavailable or vague last year might hold new meaning now. You'll read pages and sentences you don't remember. You'll be reminded of practices you forgot. Yes, these practices were written in a certain order on purpose, but now that you have a grasp of the entire process, you'll see that these practices can be done all the time and in any order. Start a new journey. Start again with this book.

I also invite you to look at the bibliography and recommended reading. These authors have inspired me on my path, and their books are excellent tools to support healing, transformation, and your yoga journey. Wisdom comes from always being teachable. Wisdom comes from understanding that we can learn an answer or solution, but the more we practice, the more natural it becomes. Inevitably, life will continue to hand us challenges, and I hope this book serves as a never-ending resource—one you can return to for ongoing comfort, support, and wisdom for whatever you are facing and wherever the path leads you.

Jai Bhagwan,
Victory to Spirit,
Molly

Acknowledgments

There are so many people involved when writing a book, especially one that chronicles a personal journey. Thank you to my yoga instructors and community at Yoga Lake Geneva in Wisconsin, who were my safe space to practice when I didn't yet know how yoga would impact my life. Thank you to Kripalu Center for Yoga and Health for imparting the wisdom of Swami Kripalu so eloquently and with such integrity so teachers and students today can benefit from yoga as both a physical and ethical practice. Thank you to AA and the recovery community for life lessons and deep friendships, which I didn't expect. Thank you to my group of supportive women writers—our monthly circles motivate and inspire me; you are the reason any book project comes to fruition. Thank you to my family and friends, who provide me with space to write through endless support and daily help. Thank you to my love, Steve, for helping me to see myself. Thank you to Angela Wix, former acquisitions editor at Llewellyn, for believing in Yoga Wise and getting it accepted for publication. Thank you to my editors, Angela and Marysa, for your valuable feedback and attention to detail.

I would like to especially thank and acknowledge all the readers of the "Monday Mantra" over the last six years. Your emails and responses about how the mantras touch, support, and encourage you have kept me writing them, and I am thrilled that they have culminated into this book.

With so much gratitude,
Molly

Recommended Reading

Bone: Dying into Life by Marion Woodman

Embodied Resilience through Yoga: 30 Mindful Essays about Finding Empowerment After Addiction, Trauma, Grief, and Loss by Kat Heagberg, Melanie C. Klein, Kathryn Ashworth, and Toni Willis

Fallen Star: A Return to Self through the Eight Limbs of Yoga by Molly Chanson

The Great Work of Your Life: A Guide for the Journey to Your True Calling by Stephen Cope

Man's Search for Meaning by Viktor E. Frankl

Not Always So: Practicing the True Spirit of Zen by Shunryū Suzuki

Outrageous Openness: Letting the Divine Take the Lead by Tosha Silver

Overcoming Trauma through Yoga: Reclaiming Your Body by David Emerson and Elizabeth Hopper

Refuge Recovery: A Buddhist Path to Recovering from Addiction by Noah Levine

A Return to Love: Reflections on the Principles of a Course in Miracles by Marianne Williamson

The Spirituality of Imperfection: Storytelling and the Search for Meaning by Ernest Kurtz and Katherine Ketcham

The Untethered Soul: The Journey Beyond Yourself by Michael A. Singer

Glossary of Sanskrit Terms

ahamkara: The I-maker, ego.

ahimsa: Nonviolence. It is the first of the five yamas.

ajna: Third eye chakra. It is the sixth chakra.

apana: Energy that flows downward in the body. It is the opposite of prana.

aparigraha: Ungrasping, to let go. It is the fifth of the five yamas.

asana: Pose.

asteya: Nonstealing. It is the third of the five yamas.

Atman: True Self.

Bhagavad Gita: A famous Hindu text that explains yoga using the story of Lord Krishna teaching his disciple, Arjuna.

Brahman: Eternal source, creator.

chitta: Mind-stuff, consciousness.

dharana: Focus. It is the sixth Limb of Yoga.

dharma: Sacred duty, soul's path.

dharmamegha: Cloud of enlightenment.

dirgha: Long.

dirgha pranayama: Three-part breath.

drishti: A single focus for sight.

granthi: Knot, doubt.

gunas: The three ropes that tie us to the material world according to Sankhya yoga philosophy.

hatha yoga: A yoga practice focused on asana and pranayama to connect body and breath.

ishvara pranidhana: Surrender to a higher power. It is the fifth of the five niyamas.

Jai Bhagwan: Victory to spirit.

japa: Mantra.

kapalabhati: Skull-shining breath.

karuna: Compassion, self-compassion.

kriya: In action, in practice.

manas: Mind.

matsyasana: Fish pose.

nadi: Energy channel.

nadi shodhana: Channel cleansing breathing.

nirodha parinama: The conjunction of the mind making a thought and the suppression of that thought.

niyama: Sacred observance. It is the second Limb of Yoga, which consists of five practices: purity and cleansing, contentment, self-discipline, self-study, and surrender.

phalakasana: Plank pose.

prakriti: Everything in nature, including matter, which is always changing.

prana: Breath, life force.

pranayama: To restrain or lengthen the breath in order to bring new awareness. It is the fourth Limb of Yoga.

pratyahara: Presence. It is the fifth Limb of Yoga.

purusha: Soul, pure consciousness.

rajas: One of the three gunas, which has qualities of fire, passion, and doing.

sadhana: Practice, realization.

samadhi: Enlightenment, liberation, and total absorption. It is the eighth Limb of Yoga.

samskara: Mental imprint.

samyogah: Union.

Sankhya: School of yoga philosophy that believes we are composed of soul (purusha) and nature (prakriti).

sattva: One of the three gunas, which has qualities of light and balance.

satya: Truth. It is the second of the five yamas.

saucha: Cleansing, purity. It is the first of the five niyamas.

shavasana: Corpse pose.

sraddha: Faith, sincerity.

tadasana: Mountain pose.

tamas: One of the three gunas, which has qualities of laziness, lethargy, and procrastination.

tapas: Self-discipline, heat, and to burn. It is the third of the five niyamas.

ugayi: Ocean-sounding breath.

vrikshasana: Tree pose.

yama: Moral restraint. It is the first Limb of Yoga, which consists of five practices: nonviolence, truth, nonstealing, nonexcess, and nongrasping, which is also called nonattachment.

yoga: Yoke, union, and practices that lead to enlightenment or liberation.

Bibliography

Adele, Deborah. *The Yamas & Niyamas: Exploring Yoga's Ethical Practice*. Duluth, MN: On-Word Bound Books, 2009.

Alcoholics Anonymous: The Story of How Many Thousands of Men and Women Have Recovered from Alcoholism. New York: Alcoholics Anonymous Worldwide Services, 2001.

Brown, Richard P., and Patricia L. Gerbarg. *The Healing Power of the Breath: Simple Techniques to Reduce Stress and Anxiety, Enhance Concentration, and Balance Your Emotions*. Boston, MA: Shambhala, 2012.

Chödrön, Pema. *When Things Fall Apart: Heart Advice for Difficult Times*. Boston, MA: Shambhala, 2016.

Chopra 21-Day Meditation Experience. "Meditation Experience." Chopra Center Meditation. https://chopracentermeditation.com.

Cope, Stephen. *The Wisdom of Yoga: A Seeker's Guide to Extraordinary Living*. New York: Bantam Books, 2007.

————. *Yoga and the Quest for the True Self.* New York: Bantam Books, 1999.

Easwaran, Eknath, trans. *The Bhagavad Gita.* Tomales, CA: Nilgiri Press, 2007.

Faulds, Richard, and Senior Teachers of Kripalu Center for Yoga & Health. *Kripalu Yoga: A Guide to Practice On and Off the Mat.* New York: Bantam Books, 2006.

Ford, Debbie. *The Dark Side of the Light Chasers: Reclaiming Your Power, Creativity, Brilliance, and Dreams.* New York: Riverhead Books, 1998.

Harris, Gabrielle. *The Language of Yin: Yoga Themes, Sequences & Inspiration to Bring Your Class to Life & Life to Your Class.* Porirua, New Zealand: Luminary Press, 2019.

Johnson, Robert A. *Owning Your Own Shadow: Understanding the Dark Side of the Psyche.* New York: Harper One, 1993.

Kingsland, James. *Siddhārtha's Brain: Unlocking the Ancient Science of Enlightenment.* New York: Harper Collins, 2016.

Kripalu Yoga Teacher Training Manual: 200-Hour Training. Stockbridge, MA: Kripalu Center for Yoga & Health, 2019.

Laframboise, Allison Gemmel, and Yoganand Michael Carroll. *Pranayama: A Path to Healing and Freedom*. Self-published, CreateSpace, 2015.

Lamott, Anne. *Bird by Bird: Some Instructions on Writing and Life*. New York: Anchor Books, 1995.

Levitt, Atma Jo Ann, ed. *Pilgrim of Love: The Life and Teachings of Swami Kripalu*. Rhinebeck, NY: Monkfish Book Publishing, 2004.

Muktibodhananda, Swami. *Hatha Yoga Pradipika: Light on Hatha Yoga*. Bihar, India: Bihar School of Yoga, 2016.

Niebuhr, Reinhold. "The Serenity Prayer and Twelve Step Recovery." Hazelden Betty Ford Foundation. Accessed August 29, 2022. https://www.hazeldenbettyford.org/articles/the-serenity-prayer.

Pagels, Elaine H. "The Gospel of Thomas." From Jesus to Christ: Frontline: PBS. Accessed August 30, 2022. https://www.pbs.org/wgbh/pages/frontline/shows/religion/story/thomas.html.

"Peace Prayer of Saint Francis." Loyola Press. Accessed August 30, 2022. https://www.loyolapress.com/catholic-resources/prayer/traditional-catholic-prayers/saints-prayers/peace-prayer-of-saint-francis/.

Satchidananda, Swami, trans. *The Yoga Sutras of Patanjali*. Yogaville, VA: Integral Yoga Publications, 2012.

Schucman, Helen, and William T. Thetford, eds. *A Course in Miracles: Workbook for Students, Manual for Teachers*. Omaha, NE: Course in Miracles Society, 2012.

Suzuki, Shunryū. *Zen Mind, Beginner's Mind*. Edited by Trudy Dixon. Boston, MA: Shambhala, 2006.

"Swami Kripalu's Inspiration for Yoga Teachers." Kripalu. Accessed January 15, 2022. https://kripalu.org/sites/default/files/kyta_quotes.pdf.

Tolle, Eckhart. *A New Earth: Awakening to Your Life's Purpose*. New York: Penguin Books, 2005.

———. *The Power of Now: A Guide to Spiritual Enlightenment*. Novato, CA: New World Library, 1999.

Tomaino, Charlotte A. *Awakening the Brain: The Neuropsychology of Grace*. New York: Atria Books, 2012.

Treleaven, David A. *Trauma-Sensitive Mindfulness: Practices for Safe and Transformative Healing*. New York: W. W. Norton & Company, 2018.

Twelve Steps and Twelve Traditions. New York: Alcoholics Anonymous World Services, 1991.

van der Kolk, Bessel A. *The Body Keeps the Score: Brain, Mind, and Body in the Healing of Trauma*. New York: Viking, 2014.

Notes

To Write to the Author

If you wish to contact the author or would like more information about this book, please write to the author in care of Llewellyn Worldwide Ltd. and we will forward your request. Both the author and the publisher appreciate hearing from you and learning of your enjoyment of this book and how it has helped you. Llewellyn Worldwide Ltd. cannot guarantee that every letter written to the author can be answered, but all will be forwarded. Please write to:

Molly Chanson, MA
^{c}/o Llewellyn Worldwide
2143 Wooddale Drive
Woodbury, MN 55125-2989

Please enclose a self-addressed stamped envelope for reply,
or $1.00 to cover costs. If outside the U.S.A., enclose
an international postal reply coupon.

Many of Llewellyn's authors have websites with additional information and resources. For more information, please visit our website at http://www.llewellyn.com.